*Medicine & Society
In America*

Medicine & Society In America

Advisory Editor

Charles E. Rosenberg
Professor of History
University of Pennsylvania

THE
MATERNAL PHYSICIAN;
A TREATISE
ON THE
NURTURE AND MANAGEMENT
OF
INFANTS,

FROM THE BIRTH UNTIL TWO YEARS OLD.

BEING THE RESULT OF

SIXTEEN YEARS' EXPERIENCE IN THE NURSERY.

ILLUSTRATED BY

EXTRACTS

FROM THE MOST APPROVED MEDICAL AUTHORS.

BY AN AMERICAN MATRON.

Introduction by
Charles E. Rosenberg

𝒜RNO 𝒫RESS & 𝒯HE 𝒩EW 𝒴ORK 𝒯IMES

New York   1972

Reprint Edition 1972 by Arno Press Inc.

Introduction Copyright © 1972 by Charles E. Rosenberg

Reprinted from a copy in
The Library of The College of
Physicians of Philadelphia

LC# 70-180581
ISBN 0-405-03958-1

Medicine and Society in America
ISBN for complete set: 0-405-03930-1
See last pages of this volume for titles.

Manufactured in the United States of America

INTRODUCTION

It seems appropriate that the female author of America's first child-care manual should be anonymous. We do not know the individual identity of the "American matron" who wrote the *Maternal Physician;* her social identity is defined by those realities of the female role with which she justified her atypical venture into authorship. By 1811, when the first edition of this little treatise appeared, she had already raised eight children, lived in the country outside Boston, and belonged to the relatively secure, servant-employing middle class. As a child she had experienced the Revolution; and at least some of her children would probably survive the Civil War. Her pages are thus particularly significant to the social historian, for they reflect the attitudes—and to an extent the experience—of a particularly formative period in American social development.

The *Maternal Physician* is most obviously a summation of the more enlightened teachings of late-eighteenth-century medicine. Though some of its admonitions are drawn from "sixteen years experience in the nursery," the basic texture of the Maternal Physician's ideas is gleaned from the most widely read English medical writers of her generation: William Buchan, Michael Underwood, Hugh Smith, and George Wallis. (All were popular in the United States; Buchan's *Domestic Medicine* and *Advice to Mothers,* for example, went through at least thirty-seven assorted American editions before 1820.) In addition to helping record the consensus of progressive medical doctrine and spell out its implications for everyday child care, the *Maternal Physician* also provides unaffected insights into popular attitudes and values. We learn, for instance, that the "lower orders" often failed to consult physicians in diseases of infancy, feeling that medicine could not help such youthful patients. Even among some of their betters, an unseemly—and to the Maternal Physician an impious—fatalism prevailed. Our anonymous author makes clear as well the roles in child rearing expected of both mother and father.

Her pages illuminate actual medical care as clearly as they do contemporary attitudes toward health and disease. We learn, for example, that women like herself still felt responsible not only for the basic health needs of their own families but also for the well-being of the poor and dependent in their vicinities. The Maternal Physician served, that is, as pediatrician and general practitioner, and she called for the physician's aid only in cases which promised to be grave indeed.

It was only natural that our author should have limited her treatise to the care of children under two, for this was conceded to be a critical age, a turning point in child development. The child had been weaned, had begun to walk and talk—hence could no longer be regarded as somehow different from older children. Equally significant in terms of contemporary medical theory, the crisis of dentition had passed. By two, moreover, our American matron assumed, the infant's character had largely been formed; it could not easily be altered in later years. The child must be treated with a mixture of affection and unwavering discipline if he was not to fall victim to "his passions and desires." The natural man was still not altogether to be trusted.

Nursing was unquestionably the most important single aspect of child care. Like many eighteenth-century child-health reformers, our American matron emphasized the importance of the mother's nursing her own child. Only in cases of death or chronic invalidism could a mother, without blame, neglect this duty and engage a wet nurse. (It must be recalled that children who were not breast-fed had only a relatively slim chance of surviving.) Both the physical and moral well-being of the child could be endangered by the improper choice of a wet nurse (for it seemed apparent that the connections forged between mother and child during nursing were of enduring importance to a child's moral and psychological, as well as physical, health). Even if the biological mother nursed her child, it was of the utmost importance that she carefully regulate her psychic and physical well-being, for stress and sickness would affect her milk and thus possibly injure the nursling who received it.

Even if a child weathered the period of nursing without injury, he still had to endure the crisis of dentition. Like puberty and menopause, teething was considered one of those periodic developmental crises which had to be withstood if prospects for health in later life were not to be damaged. A proper diet, fresh air, exercise, and amusement were necessary if the infant body was to emerge from dentition unscarred. Even in apparently quite healthy infants, moreover, teething might bring dangerous fevers or wasting dysentery. To facilitate the process and relieve the physiological stress which caused such ills, the Maternal Physician strongly urged routine lancing of the gums with a sharp razor.

Following the reformist admonitions of her favorite medical authors, the Maternal Physician reiterated the need for a "natural" regimen. Cleanliness, freedom in dress, the opportunity to exercise, and a wholesome moderation in diet were all essential to ensuring continued good health. The swaddling bands, heavy clothing, stays, and walking stools which constrained children of previous generations were now to be discarded. The infant must not be allowed to remain in filth. Dirt was more dangerous than drafts; his every morning should begin with a cold bath. The Maternal Physician's attitude toward drugs, though moderate for her generation, can hardly be considered nihilistic. She urged the routine use of mild laxatives—even in dysentery. If a child experienced difficulty in sleeping through the night, it seemed better to provide some paregoric or poppies than allow discomfort to continue unabated—though such measures should not, she warned, be allowed to become routine as they had in many homes.

But it is hardly necessary to reiterate in detail the cautions and admonitions our anonymous author has so lucidly presented. To an extraordinary extent, this little *vade mecum* speaks for itself: the necessarily recurring realities of the human experience providing an appropriate entree to her concerns and anxieties. Perhaps, indeed, it is her acceptance of the responsibilities inherent in woman's traditional role which is most striking to the twentieth-century sensibility. To be a wife and mother in the New Republic was to accept fear, danger, and pain as conditions of life. Though childbirth meant "agonies almost insupportable," the Maternal Physician sought shrewdly to make those women who survived better and more enlightened mothers, mothers fit for the needs of a vigorous new nation.

Charles E. Rosenberg
University of Pennsylvania
October, 1972

THE
MATERNAL PHYSICIAN;
A TREATISE
ON THE
NURTURE AND MANAGEMENT
OF
INFANTS,

FROM THE BIRTH UNTIL TWO YEARS OLD.

BEING THE RESULT OF

SIXTEEN YEARS' EXPERIENCE IN THE NURSERY.

ILLUSTRATED BY

EXTRACTS

FROM THE MOST APPROVED MEDICAL AUTHORS.

BY AN AMERICAN MATRON.

"Light were my task if every gentle breast
"Owned the just laws of native truth imprest;
"For not by hopes of vain applause misled,
"In reason's injured cause alone I plead.
"'Tis yours to judge; nor I that judgment fear,
"If truth be sacred, and if virtue dear."
Roscoe, from the Italian of Luigi Transillo.

SECOND EDITION.

PHILADELPHIA:
PUBLISHED BY LEWIS ADAMS.
Clark & Raser, Printers.
1818.

District of New York, ss.

BE IT REMEMBERED, That on the sixth day of August, in the thirty-sixth year of the independence of the United States of America, ISAAC RILEY, of the said district, hath deposited in this office the title of a book, the right whereof he claims as proprietor, in the words following, to wit:

" The Maternal Physician; a Treatise on the Nurture and Management of Infants, from the birth until two years old. Being the result of sixteen years experience in the Nursery. Illustrated by Extracts from the most approved Medical Authors. By an American Matron.

" Light were my task if every gentle breast
" Owned the just laws of native truth imprest;
" For not by hopes of vain applause misled,
" In reason's injured cause alone I plead.
" 'Tis yours to judge; nor I that judgment fear,
" If truth be sacred, and if virtue dear."
Roscoe, from the Italian of Luigi Transillo.

In conformity to the act of the congress of the United States, entitled, " An act for the encouragement of learning, by securing the copies of maps, charts, and books, to the authors and proprietors of such copies, during the times therein mentioned."— And also to the act, entitled, " An act supplementary to an act, entitled, ' An act for the encouragement of learning, by securing the copies of maps, charts, and books, to the authors and proprietors of such copies during the times therein mentioned,' and extending the benefits thereof to the arts of designing, engraving, and etching historical and other prints."

CHARLES CLINTON,
Clerk of the District of New York.

DEDICATION.

TO MY MOTHER.

MADAM,

THAT helpless babe which reposed on your affrighted bosom when you fled the vicinity of Boston, on the day of the ever memorable battle of Lexington, now a wife, a mother, and near the meridian of life, as a small tribute for all your maternal cares, most respectfully addresses this little volume to your perusal; candidly confessing that all which is valuable in it she derived from you.

For the nurture of my infancy I am most grateful—but for my education, and, above all, for the sublime lesson you taught me, *" that the best pleasures of a woman's life are found in the faithful discharge of her maternal duties,"* I owe you more than gratitude.

May you find an ample recompense in the assurance that from your grandchildren I receive that filial love and respect which has ever been rendered you by

Your Daughter

MARY.

INTRODUCTION.

EVERY MOTHER HER CHILD'S BEST PHYSICIAN.

Some time since, while looking over a file of old newspapers, I cast my eyes upon the obituaries, and was forcibly impressed with the great proportion of children who are yearly consigned to the relentless grave under the age of two years. I revolved in my mind why it was so, and could not avoid concluding that it must be in a great measure occasioned by some gross mismanagement in mothers or nurses, or perhaps in both. Involuntarily I looked around upon my own children, and my heart swelled with gratitude to heaven for hitherto averting the shafts of the fell destroyer from them, and permitting the roses of health to bloom on their cheeks with almost uninterrupted continuity.

Deeply impressed by this invaluable blessing of a merciful Providence, I felt an irresistible desire to see the same felicity pervade every maternal bosom. But alas! imagination presented to my view the sick or the dying babe, and the anxious or distracted mother, and I ardently wished to extend my hand, feeble though it might be, to their relief. And why, thought I, may not this be done. I remembered, when my first child was an infant, how easily I was alarmed if he was ill, and how eagerly I caught at every glimpse of light that promised to direct me in the management of him; I recollected the words of an eminent physician, whom I was in the habit of summoning every time my babe looked paler than usual. "You may yourself be your child's best physician," said this excellent man, "if you only will attend to a few general directions." I promised faithful obedience; and Heaven has crowned my endeavours with success: why then may I not show my gratitude, by presenting to the matrons of my country the fruits of my experience, in the pleasing hope that I may be instrumental in directing them in the all-important and delightful task of nursing those sweet pledges of connubial love, over whom every good mother watches with tremulous anxiety, and almost painful affection. A very near and dear friend, not entirely unknown in the literary world, approving my plan, I have resolved on the attempt, and if I can happily aid in preserving but one lovely babe from fell disease, in averting the deadliest arrow of affliction from the bosom of but one mother, great will be my reward. I am well aware how much has been written on this subject by the most able physicians, to whom I acknowledge myself indebted for many useful hints; but these gentlemen must pardon me if I think, after all, that a mother is her child's best physician, in all ordinary cases; and that none but a mother can tell how to *nurse* an infant as it ought to be nursed. Who but a mother can possibly feel interest enough in a helpless new born babe to pay it that unwearied, uninterrupted attention necessary to detect in season any latent symptoms of disease lurking in its tender frame, and which, if neglected, or injudiciously treated at first, might in a few hours baffle the physician's skill, and consign it to the grave?

And believe me, my fair friends, this is not a labour. What can so sweetly relieve the tedium of three or four weeks' confinement to a sick room, as to watch with unremitting care, and mark with enraptured eye, the opening beauties of the dear innocent cause of such confinement? Or what can equal a mother's ecstasy when she catches the first emanation of mind in the mantling smile of her babe? Kotzebue little knew the mother's heart when he makes Cora place her first joy after birth, "When first the white blossoms of his teeth appear, breaking the crimson buds that did encase them." Ten thousand raptures thrill her bosom before a tooth is formed. How dead to the finest feelings of our nature must that mother be, who can voluntarily banish her infant from her bosom, and thus forego the exquisite delight attending the first development of its rational faculties. O fashion! arbitrary tyrant, of what hours of heartfelt bliss dost thou deprive thy votary—

> " One lovely babe *her* fostering care demands;
> " And can *she* trust it to a hireling's hands?"

Far distant, I trust, from our beloved country,

is the period when it shall be accounted disgraceful for a mother to nurse her own babe. When that time arrives my system must fall to the ground. It is upon the presumption, that my readers are among those who glory in the sweetest privilege of nature, and are never more blest

> " Than whilst their babe, with unpolluted lips,
> " As nature asks, the vital fountain sips."

that I presume to offer my advice; for it is under such circumstances only that a mother can observe all the minutiæ of her child's state of health.

Experience has taught me that the babe who was to all appearance well in the morning may droop in the afternoon, be very ill at night, and yet, by proper care and attention, again be well the next morning; when, perhaps, the same babe if neglected or improperly treated, would have been seized with fits, or some equally fatal complaint, and possibly have died in less time. For the truth of this statement, I appeal to those who are skilled in those dreadful disorders the quinsy and the croup. It is upon cases similar to this, that I ground my hypothesis that every mother is her child's best physician; and how can a mother reconcile her conscience when she consigns this precious little being, given her by Providence to be her comfort through life, and the staff of her declining age, to the care of a stranger, when assured that one day's neglect might deprive her of it for ever, and blast her fondest hopes.

> " Ah then, by duty led, ye nuptial fair,
> " Let the sweet office be your constant care;
> " With peace and health in humblest station blest,
> " Give to the smiling babe the fostering breast;
> " Nor if by prosperous fortune placed on high,
> " Think aught superior to the dear employ."
> " Not half a mother she, whose pride denies
> " The streaming beverage to her infant's cries,
> " Admits another in her rights to share,
> " Or trusts its nurture to a stranger's care."

That there are many instances when the mother's health will not permit her to suckle her child I will allow; but I must believe those cases would less frequently occur if the attempt were persevered in. This I assert from experience in one remarkable instance. My first child had the thrush when about a fortnight old. I had previously suffered great pain from an exuberant flow of milk, and was greatly weakened by it. Now I took the humour from his mouth, and for two months he seldom sucked without throwing up fresh blood afterwards, which he had swallowed with his milk. The torture I endured can better be conceived than described. Many of my friends with tears entreated me to wean my child, and dry away my milk, which, owing to loss of appetite and fever, occasioned by excess of suffering, might then have been done with ease; but my own mother, who watched over me and my babe with more than maternal tenderness, and who, I am convinced, felt all I suffered with redoubled anguish, constantly exhorted me to persevere with fortitude, nor let any thing I endured tempt me to tear my babe from the breast, and by improper food occasion ill health, if not endanger his life; for amidst all my distress I had the inexpressible delight of seeing him thrive surprisingly. I listened to my mother, for my judgment was on her side, and had abundant cause to rejoice that I did so, for the days of affliction passed away as a dream, and left the sweet consciousness of having done my duty as a recompense for suffering; a recompense, how rich, how lasting, how consoling! Had I weakly yielded in the hour of pain, and dried away my milk, it is more than probable, from the bad state the humours were then in, some unnatural contractions would have taken place, and not only that child but all my succeeding family would have suffered from it. Therefore I entreat every mother to undergo every thing short of death or lasting disease, rather than refuse to suckle her child. There are now many useful inventions for drawing out the milk, which were not in general use when I was so afflicted; and if it can be drawn out with sucking glasses, and the babe fed with it for a few days in cases similar to the one related above, it will without doubt be far better both for mother and child: upon this plan the milk may be preserved; for it is a fact, that while the babe is nourished by it, it will continue to flow, let it be obtained from the breast how it may; whereas, if it is drawn out and thrown away, the mother will have less and less until it eventually dries away entirely.* It may not be amiss to mention here, for the benefit of the afflicted, that the remedy I eventually found most efficacious in this distressing complaint was *white lead*. After trying various applications, and employing several physicians, in vain, this was acciden-

---

* This statement may perhaps excite a smile of incredulity in the learned reader, because the fact cannot be accounted for on any known principles. Facts, however, are not made by theory, but theory created by facts. If the fact that a mother's milk will cease to flow when it is thrown away, and continue to flow when given to her babe, is derided by the learned, it will only meet the fate of discoveries every way more important. The same thing has always happened. An operation of nature is noticed by the vulgar: if the learned cannot account for it, those who credit it are derided as weak and credulous, and its existence is denied; but when it can be no longer denied, the learned set down seriously to account for it; they publish their reveries; and this is called theory. The sneer of derision is then on the other side; and those who do not at once admit the fact and the theory, are ranked among the weak and the vulgar. I believe in the existence of *this* fact; and if it can derive support from analogy, I appeal to every observing dairy woman if the same does not happen in the management of her milch-kine.

tally recommended by a lady who had herself experienced the same affliction. The cooling qualities of the ceruse appeared to allay the distressing heat of the humour, and, by its absorbency to heal and sooth the part. Great care, however, must be taken when using it, carefully to wash the breast with warm milk and water before the child is permitted to suck.

But if, after all, my amiable friends, you should actually be so unhappy as to be obliged to permit your infant to draw its first nourishment from a stranger, let me advise you to have your nurse under your own roof if possible. Notwithstanding all the horrors so poetically described in an elegant little poem already quoted in the preceding pages, called "The Nurse," translated from the Italian by that learned and fascinating writer, William Roscoe, of Liverpool, (and which I would recommend to the perusal of every lady who hesitates for a moment whether to nurse her infant herself or not, from a blind devotedness to fashion, or still more reprehensible indolence of disposition,) if your babe is in the house with you, you can with ease pay it every attention requisite to its health, and thus discharge the only remaining duty in your power. You can observe, and by your authority oblige your nurse to observe, the state of its bowels, and other indications of disease.

> " Sick, pale and languid, when your infant's moans
> " Speaks its soft sufferings in pathetic tones,
> " When nature asks a purer lymph, subdued
> " By needful physic and by temperate food,"

it must be your care to see the proper regimen adopted and medicine taken. You will also have it in your power to prevent the attendants from crowding its little stomach with pap and other crudities, which I fear are too often given, from a mistaken tenderness, to the great injury of the child. You will likewise be able to watch that your babe is not exposed to every change of atmosphere. I have known a fine healthy child seized with a violent quinsy, owing to carelessness in exposing it to the evening air after a sultry day. Indifferent persons are apt to forget that an infant in arms, from inactivity, is much more sensible of the cold than those who attend it, who from that very exertion keep up a brisk circulation of the blood, which renders them less obnoxious to the deleterious effects of any sudden change in the air. For this reason a mother is her child's best physician, as it is better by care to prevent disease, than to be ever so well skilled in curing it.

> " Once exiled from your breast, and doomed to bring
> " His daily nurture from a stranger spring,
> " Ah who can tell the dangers that await
> " Your infant, thus abandoned to his fate?"

Let your tenderness, then, render you tremblingly alive to every appearance of danger. Do not, however, imagine, from what is here said, that I mean to advocate a too delicate regimen for infants. The following pages, if they respond to my wishes, will fully prove the contrary. I only wish such care to be taken of them, as their extreme tenderness evidently demands. If a child is properly and faithfully nursed the first year, it will have gained such a portion of health and strength by that time, as will enable it to bear all the exercise in the open air which its age will admit; and then the more it is carried abroad the better. when the weather is fair. When

> " The rural wilds
> " Invite; the mountains call you, and the vales,

" The woods, the streams, and each ambrosial breeze
" That fans the ever undulating sky;
" A kindly sky! whose fostering power regales
" Man, beast, and all the vegetable reign."

ARMSTRONG.

Eight lovely and beloved children, who have all (except the three youngest) passed through the usual epidemics of our country, and now enjoy an unusual proportion of health and strength, are the best apologies I can offer for thus presuming to give my advice unasked, and perhaps undesired, to my fair countrywomen. The motive, I trust, will insure my pardon for any traits of egotism, which must unavoidably appear while recommending a mode of treatment founded chiefly upon my own experience; but which, nevertheless, the better to enforce, I intend to enrich with casual extracts from the most approved medical authorities.

In the following work I propose to take the babe from the birth, and attend it through every stage until it is two years old; after which period children in general, having cut all their teeth, grow more robust, (that is, if they have been properly managed,) and will increase in health and strength without any attention except the ordinary care conducive to cleanliness and exercise, two points never to be dispensed with through life.

That I may not tire your patience, and in the pleasing hope that from what has been said, you will be inclined to believe a mother *may* be her child's best physician, if she is desirous to be so, I shall now proceed to my first chapter, in which I shall endeavour to enable her to manage her babe from the birth until it is four months old; the time when they generally begin to breed teeth, and consequently require an appropriate treatment. And I do verily believe, if the directions I shall give are faithfully attended to, many a fond mother will have reason to rejoice in the experiment.

> " Think not that I would bid your softness share
> " Undue fatigue, and every grosser care;
> " Another's toils may here supply your own,
> " But be the task of *nurture* yours alone;
> " Nor from a stranger let your offspring prove
> " The fond endearments of a parent's love—
> " So shall your child in manhood's riper day,
> " With warm affection all your cares repay."

CHESNUT HILL,
  June, 1810.

THE

MATERNAL PHYSICIAN.

CHAPTER I.

SECTION I.

On the proper Treatment of Infants, under the Age of four Months.

"For thee health gushes from a thousand springs." Pope.

I NEED not attempt to describe the rapture that swells a mother's heart, when, after agonies almost insupportable, her babe is given to her arms. Every mother knows that language is inadequate to such a description. It is perhaps equally impossible to paint her anxiety to preserve a life so dearly bought, so highly valued; or with what fervent devotion she lifts her soul to *Him* who gave it, in supplications for its health and safety. In the sweet yet humble hope of contributing towards an end so desirable, I shall attempt to exhibit in the following pages the fruits of sixteen years' unremitted attention to the complaints, the wants, the tempers, dispositions, and desires of children. And when I assure my readers that I have nursed all my children myself, and have been their constant attendant in sickness and in health, they will allow me to have had a competent share of experience. In this long course of observation I have become convinced that if the simple method I shall recommend was generally adopted, the lives of thousands would be saved, and many a fond parent's heart escape the reiterated "sting of death" in the persons of their children—

———"a consummation
Devoutly to be wished"—

in the accomplishment of which no pains should be spared; no means left unessayed. Good nursing, especially cleanliness, is among the first things to be considered. Therefore, after a new born babe has undergone the usual washing with warm suds, made with Castile, or other purified soap, let it be carefully washed with *cold water ;* not immersed.

for that appears to me, a cruel and unnecessary practice; but let the nurse have ready a basin of cold water, and with a warm hand wash the infant's head, face, neck, behind its ears, under the arms, the legs, feet, in the groin, and every part peculiarly subject to excoriation; she must then have a warm soft cloth, and wipe it perfectly dry as quick as possible, and proceed to dress it, as usual. Particular attention should be paid to wiping it, for if the water is left in the creases of the neck or elsewhere, it may do more hurt than good, by increasing their natural liability to chafe and become sore. This washing I would have repeated every morning, with this exception, that after the first dressing the cold water will be sufficient. Do not, I entreat you, my fair friends, from a mistaken tenderness, reject this salutary practice. We are acknowledged creatures of habit; and when the cold bathing is thus used from the birth, infants in general will soon become pleased with it. I have now a fine boy, scarce four months old, who was born in the winter, when the weather was most inclement; yet this did not deter me from insisting upon his being thoroughly washed with cold water before he was dressed ; and the practice has never been omitted a single day since ; and now he will spring to the basin, evidently wishing to put his hands in the water, and laugh while it trickles down his neck. Many good women have called me cruel, and protested it was unnatural thus to deluge a poor little innocent with cold water ; asserting that a little spirit of any kind was much better. Now I would ask which is the most cruel or unnatural ; to lave its little limbs with the pure element, designed by a beneficent Creator for our purification, and consequent health, and beauty ; or with ardent spirits, which, when applied to the skin of a new born babe, already perhaps in many places excoriated, must occasion intolerable smarting and pain. Let an experiment for once be tried of each, and the child by its cries will quickly decide to which it gives the preference. However, if an infant continues, after a few days, to show an uncommon aversion to the cold bath, I would by no means insist upon perfectly cold water ; in such cases it may be rendered tepid. I remember one of my children never would submit to washing with cold water, without screaming violently, and to this day, when he is six years old, has an unaccountable dread of it; but remember this is only one out of eight, and he has been the most unwell of any of my family. I do not say this is owing to my indulgence in substituting the tepid for the cold bath; perhaps it was some constitutional infirmity which rendered him from his birth so averse to it. The great desideratum, cleanliness, may be achieved in either way; but still I beg leave to repeat my earnest request that the cold water may be faithfully tried; it invigorates the system, renders the babe strong and healthy, and, by preventing irritation and soreness, permits it to sleep quietly, which every new born child inclines to do when not prevented by pain.

SECTION II.

"Each thing that fitted gentleness to wear." DRAYTON.

To aid this natural desire and evident necessity of rest, the dress of so young an infant cannot be too light and easy; but in our inclement climate some regard must be paid to the season of the year. In winter the more flannel is substituted for other materials in their clothing, the better ; it greatly contributes to their comfort and health. As a general rule, I think their usual dress may be in this season, a foot blanket of fine flannel, a petticoat of the same, and a frock of any material the mother may fancy ; these, with a cap and shirt of the lightest materials possible, are quite sufficient for every purpose of health and comfort. If the season is approaching to summer, I would omit the flannel coat, and let its place be supplied with one of a lighter texture, preserving the foot blanket as better calculated to wrap around the feet ; and every mother knows, if she attends to her child, that the moment its feet are cold it seems to be in pain, and that it is quieted again by warming them by the fire, or in any other way. An infant's feet should never be exposed to the cold air ; at the same time it ought not to be loaded with clothes, to increase its natural propensity to perspiration. Perhaps it were better to wrap a light flannel mantle about the babe occasionally, which might with ease be thrown off, as the weather grew warm, rather than encumber its little frame with too much clothing the first month or six weeks. Care must nevertheless be taken not to err on the other hand. A judicious writer observes, "*Infants should always be cool, but never cold.*"* But what I esteem of still more essential consequence, and would particularly enforce, is *changing* an infant's clothes frequently. I would choose it should be done every day. I know many ladies who are perfectly correct on this head; but I likewise

---

* *Michael Underwood*, M. D. Licentiate in Midwifery, of the Royal College of Physicians in London, Physician to her Royal Highness, the Princess of Wales, and Senior Physician to the British Lying-in Hospital, in a Treatise on the Diseases of Children and Management of Infants from the Birth; a book perused with much pleasure and profit by the author of this work, and warmly recommended to her fair readers. For, perhaps, after making due allowance for certain positions, in the assuming of which he was obliged to pay homage to the high bred prejudices of a luxurious city and age, there are few European medical writers who can be read with so much advantage, as applicable to the diseases or management of infants in the United States.

know many affectionate mothers, who err greatly from a mistaken fear of making their children take cold. Believe me, there is no danger of this, provided the clothes are perfectly well aired. A child should never be suffered to sleep in any part of the dress worn during the day ; for besides the most indispensable object in nursing, cleanliness, many other advantages accrue to the infant from thus often dressing and undressing it; it gives the mother or nurse frequent opportunities to examine the whole body, and by that means discover any excoriation or chafing. Opening it to the air before the fire, (if the weather requires one,) and rubbing its little limbs, gives a spring to the blood, invigorates the frame, and inclines it to stretch, which facilitates the growth and beauty of its form. Every mother should reflect upon the great utility of promoting the kindly circulation of the fluids, and keeping open the pores,

>"The grand discharge, th' effusion of the skin
>"Slowly impaired, the languid maladies
>"Creep on, and through the sinking functions steal."
>
>ARMSTRONG.

And what can so greatly contribute to both

these requisites as the method here recommended. To those mothers, however, who, from early prejudice, or any other cause, should object to putting fresh clothes upon their child every day, permit me to suggest the propriety of having an entire night suit, even to the shirt, and entreat them to see that their babes are carefully examined all over every night and morning, and gently rubbed in all parts of the body, especially the back. In this way the clothing may be constantly kept smooth about them, and any eruption or other complaint detected in season, the necessity of which is sufficiently obvious. Dr. Buchan, in his Family Physician, mentions a child who died in convulsion fits, and after it was dead a pin was discovered thrust half its length or more into the body of the little sufferer; which he thinks was the only cause of the fits, and consequently of its death! My blood recoils with horror while I think of the wretched mother when she made this discovery; may it be a solemn warning to every one who has the care of an infant to carefully search for some such cause when their helpless little charge by its cries makes the only complaint in its power.

> "What ceaseless dread a mother's breast alarms
> "Whilst her loved offspring fills another's arms!
> "Fearful of ill, she starts at every noise,
> "And hears, or thinks she hears, her children's cries."

One thing more should be mentioned here, which, as I esteem of very essential consequence, although entirely neglected by many, I shall beg leave (lest my authority should be disputed) to notice in the words of Dr. Buchan.

"Combing the heads of infants should by no means be neglected; they are apt to acquire a kind of scurf beneath the hair, which stops the pores, and is productive of headach and weak eyes; to which, from a mere omission of this useful operation, most young children are subject. But a fine comb, and very tender hand, are requisite in the performance of this task." For this reason I never suffer any hand but my own to perform it for my children while at this early age.

And now, as I have said all that I think necessary as to the washing and clothing of infants, I will proceed to the still more important point, *their food*.

SECTION III.

The Mother's Milk the best and only proper Food for Infants.

"Doubt ye the laws by nature's God ordained?
"Or that the callow young should be sustained
"Upon the parent breast? be those your schools
"Where nature triumphs and where instinct rules."

NEW born infants, if well, (as they generally are at the birth,) require no food but what they will obtain from the mother's breast; and if ill, peculiar care should be taken not to crowd their little stomachs with any improper mixtures. I am well aware that this doctrine will be rejected by many who believe it absolutely necessary to give the little creatures some nauseous draught or other, to promote the natural evacuations. But trust me this is a great mistake; and be persuaded to accept as proof my own experience. As soon as my children are dressed, I always order them to be brought to me, and put them immediately to the breast. O what a blissful moment to a fond mother! when

> "The starting beverage meets the thirsty lip,
> "'Tis joy to yield it, and 'tis joy to sip;"

and I never had the least occasion to use any other medicine for my babes. But if my authority is not sufficient, hear what **Dr. Buchan** says upon the subject.

"Children commonly show a disposition to suck very shortly after the birth, and they should unquestionably be immediately indulged, if the mother's milk begins to flow into the breast; and should it be slow in its progress, the natural industry of the infant will speedily supply the deficiency. The first milk it can draw is the best medicine in the world to cleanse its little stomach and bowels of the matter acquired in the womb; and at the same time contributes to the safety of the mother, by preventing milk fevers, inflammations, and other complaints incident to women in childbed."

It is true it will not at first obtain much; but it will ordinarily get enough to support it until the milk comes, which (as observed by the judicious author just quoted) will be very soon, when thus gently invited by the sweetest call of nature. It is well known that when a child is not put to the breast until the milk is fully come; which in that case is seldom until the third or fourth day, it must be fed: this unnatural food clogs the first passages, occasions acidities, wind, and their usual distressing consequences; recourse is then had to oils, syrups, and even spirituous liquors, which greatly increase the irritation. In this state the poor little babe is at length permitted to suck inordinately from a full breast of milk, while the mother herself is feverish and ill from the sudden change her system has undergone : the fatal effects may be easily imagined; and who can wonder if children so managed are frequently seized with convulsions, and die within a few days. Therefore let me entreat you to take your infants to your bosom immediately, and leave Nature to do her own work, in which, as it respects so material a point as providing food for her offspring, it is almost presumptuous to think her deficient.

It will sometimes happen, however, that from some unknown cause a new born infant evinces such indisputable signs of hunger as it would be cruel to disregard. If, therefore, after the babe has drawn all it can obtain from its mother, (which for its medicinal qualities it should be allowed to do as soon as possible) it should still show indications of hunger, such as eagerly sucking its fingers, and then crying from disappointment, it should be permitted to suck some healthy woman with a good breast of milk. It is almost superfluous to observe that the younger such milk may be, the more salubrious it must prove for so young an infant. And if it should be impossible to find a woman with convenience who could give it the breast, it may be fed with a little good cow's milk, diluted with nearly half water, and rendered palatable with sugar. After this first craving is allayed, the child will fall asleep, and afterwards be perfectly satisfied with what it can obtain from its mother. Too much food occasions acidities and griping in such young children; oftener the cause of their crying, and infinitely more hurtful to them than the temporary want of food they may feel previous to the full flowing of the milk, even allowing that they do feel such want, which I believe rarely happens, provided they are permitted to suck as often as they show a disposition to do so. Here, I suppose, I shall have the disciples of the late Dr. Hugh Smith to combat. Through a mistaken complaisance to ladies of over-refined delicacy, and with a laudable wish to persuade them that they may *possibly* undergo the fatigue of nursing their own children, that gentleman has attempted to prove, in his letters to married women, that the meals of an infant may be regulated like those of adults, and that if they are suffered to suck four or five times in four and twenty hours, it is sufficient. I will not say this cannot be done, but I will say I would not for any consideration undertake to bring up a little babe from the birth so hampered. I have often been vexed with physicians who, while they exhort us to follow nature, from a misplaced indulgence to the prevailing fastidiousness of the age, adopt the absurd notion that a mother cannot endure the fatigue of suckling her own child. This may be the case in some few instances. Such unhappy mothers are to be pitied, but I greatly fear the far greater number who neglect this sweet endearing office are more fit objects of censure than pity.

Any woman, how delicate soever her education and habits, who is capable of becoming the mother of a child, may nurse it if she pleases, unless prevented by illness; and indeed she whom education has rendered thus delicate is doubly reprehensible for neglecting this prime maternal duty; as it is to be presumed Providence has given her the means of providing herself every assistance necessary, and every indulgence even to superfluity.

How ungrateful to that benign Providence, thus to turn the greatest blessings into evils the most lamentable, and by giving way to a sickly delicacy, and fashions and opinions totally repugnant to the finest feelings of the soul, cast from her fostering bosom the sweet pledge of her heart's best affections, and expose it to sickness and sorrow, if not to *death.*

> " But you whose hearts with gentle pity warm,
> " Pure joys can please and genuine pleasures charm,
> " Clasp your fair nurslings to your breasts of snow,
> " And give the sweet salubrious streams to flow;
> " Let kind affections sway without control,
> " And through the milk-streams pour the feeling soul."

But to return to my subject: as it is above every thing desirable to keep the infant quiet, both because crying is the occasion of ruptures in such young children, and that the mother and babe mutually require rest, it may be better to feed it occasionally with the milk and water rather than let it complain for want of food; but do not on any account suffer your attendants to cram its little stomach with pap, or any other thick food. I shall here beg leave to insert an extract from a work I have read with great benefit and pleasure. Speaking of the great folly of feeding infants with what the author calls " thick victuals," he says—

" On this article a vast crowd of absurdities open upon us at once, and many of them with the sanction of custom and authority. I shall first advert to the thickness of the food: and it has, indeed, been a matter of wonder, how the custom of stuffing new born infants with bread could become so universal, or the idea first enter the mind of a parent, that such heavy food could be fit for its nourishment. It were well if the fond mother, and all well-inclined nurses, had more just ideas of the manner in which we are nourished; and especially, that it is not from the great quantity, nor from the quality of the food, abstractedly considered; since the inhabitants of different parts of the globe are equally healthy and long-lived who feed upon the most opposite diets. Parents, one should think, may very easily conceive that our nourishment arises from the use the stomach makes of the food it receives; which is to pass through such a change called digestion, as renders it balsamic, and fit to renew the mass of blood which is daily wasting and consumed. An improper kind, or too great a quantity taken at a time, or too hastily, before the stomach has duly disposed of its former contents, prevents this work of digestion, and, by making bad juices, weakens instead of strengthens the habit; and in the end produces worms, convulsions, rickets, kings-evil, slow fevers, purging, and general decay.

" Nature, it should be considered, has provided only milk for every animal adapted to draw it from the breast, and that of women is certainly among the thinnest of them; but at the same time, far more nutritive than bread, and, probably, than any other milk, as it contains a greater proportion of saccharine matter, which is thought to be that quality in all our food which renders it nutritious. It is true, bread, as it requires more digestion, will lie longer on the stomach both of infants and adults; and hence, probably, because it satisfies the present cravings, it has been conceived to afford a greater proportion of nourishment: though mixed up only with water, as it too frequently is, it is far less nutritive than has been imagined; for the water affords no nourishment, and the bread is but imperfectly digested. Children ought to be frequently hungry, and as often supplied with light food, of which milk is really the most nourishing we are acquainted with."

From authority so indisputable I presume there will be no appeal. Therefore, as I wish to enable my fair readers to manage the infants committed to their care without being obliged to call in a physician for every trifling indisposition, I will now beg leave briefly to notice such little complaints as are generally incident to them at this early age; with the remedies I have from long experience found

D

beneficial. I shall also, as mentioned in my introduction, occasionally enforce my opinions with the best medical authorities, lest some fond mothers should doubt my ability to direct on so important an occasion as where the health, and, possibly, the lives, of their children are concerned. Honouring, as I most cordially do, every indication of maternal tenderness, I reverence even prejudices arising from so amiable a source; and therefore, as I proceed, I shall endeavour to obviate such as I think most injurious to the health of infants, by arguments drawn from the best authorities, as well as from my own successful experience, rather than by asserting them to be either false or unfounded.

SECTION IV.

On Diseases incident to the Navel.

" To watch the infant form with anxious care,
" The lurking symptoms of disease detect,
" And with the aid of sweet nutritious food,
" Or potent herb, or kindly drug, to aid
" Oppressed nature in her arduous task
" Be thine! and thine the grateful rich reward
" Of conscious duty done—a mead more fair
" Than all the laurels which bedeck the brow
" Of modern Cæsar."

As this is a part which requires the earliest attention, and which, as every nurse knows, will call for particular care the first fortnight of the infant's existence, and sometimes much longer, I shall notice it here. It is not my intention, however, to enter into the treatment of ruptures, or any other uncommon disorder of this part which may possibly occur, as every mother in such cases would undoubtedly wish for the best professional aid and advice. I shall confine myself to the common complaints, and the best method of treating them, that has come within my knowledge. As young mothers and nurses are sometimes at a loss how to proceed in the first dressing of the child, it may perhaps be advantageous to insert a quotation from Dr. Buchan upon that subject in the first place. "If too much of the cord or navel string is left to the body of the child, it is apt to occasion inflammation; nay, in some cases, even mortification. The best way of managing it is, to make a hole in a piece of fine linen, many times doubled, and passing the end of the navel string through the hole, to fold the cloth several times till it gets near the belly; to which it should be bound by a smooth roller (or belly-band) but not drawn too tight. The navel string commonly separates and falls off in four or five days; when that happens, which should be carefully attended to, a bit of singed rag may be laid over the navel; and if any rawness or soreness should appear round it, and the skin should be fretted or galled, a raisin split and stoned may be applied, and the part washed with a little alum water, or a weak solution of sugar of lead, and a plaster of cerate applied, to protect it from rubbing." I have always been in the habit of roasting the raisin, and grating upon it a little nutmeg; and I think the dressing ought to be renewed every day, and the part anointed with sweet oil in preference to the waters recommended above. I observe that Dr. Underwood enters largely into the treatment of this part, and to his book I would refer all those who wish for more particular information. But as some of my readers may not have it either in their power or inclination to consult so large a work, I will for their convenience extract from it what is said upon the most common complaints incident to it at this age.

" A complete separation (of the cord) in some instances takes place in five days, and even earlier; and in others not until the fifteenth or sixteenth. When so late, the cord is usually found to hang for some time only by a very small filament or thread, which, having no life remaining, ought to be divided. For want of this a source of irritation and discharge is kept up, which I have suspected being the cause of some of the little disorders of this part. The separation, however, is not often followed with much soreness or pain though there is frequently a true ulcer of the part. In some instances, however, the discharge is very great, and the part continues to appear raw and indisposed to heal or dry up. In such cases, I have often found three or four small pieces of a soft cabbage leaf one of the best applications. They should be laid one over another, that they may be preserved moist and cool, and should be continued as long as the discharge shall be considerable." I have had one instance among my children similar to the one last mentioned, and found a plaster of Turner's cerate the best application among a variety I made use of. Parents are often alarmed at the protrusion of the navel, mistaking it for a rupture, but as that rarely happens, great care should be taken not to attempt reducing it by any violent means. The best way of avoiding such alarming appearances is to suffer the child to wear the belly-band at least six weeks, provided the weather is not extremely warm; and when it is removed, directions should be given to its attendant to press the hand firmly but gently upon that part, if the child should chance to cry violently. The vulgar opinion that a large navel is the sign of a crying child, is a conclusive argument in favour of the above precaution.

Red Gum, or Benign Eruption.

THIS is a complaint (if it can be called one) incident I believe to every child, and therefore perfectly well known. It has probably obtained the name of *Benign Eruption* from its being a sign of health in the child, when it appears profusely on the surface. It usually appears in the course of the first week in the form of a fine rash, first upon the neck and the inside of the arms and about the face, from whence it generally spreads to every part of the body in spots, particularly those parts which are the most covered. It usually continues upon the surface two or three weeks, and will sometimes appear again at intervals until the child is six weeks or two months old. When it first appears, it is best to give the babe a little saffron tea to assist in throwing it out, and defend the stomach in case it should suddenly disappear, which, however, will seldom happen, if the child is managed from the birth according to the preceding directions; care also being taken to keep it from the cold. Little or no medicine is required except to keep the body open. If the infant is costive, small doses of rhubarb and magnesia may be given in a little of any of the warming or aromatic waters, such as mint or carraway; if these are not to be had, common water will do. My last child, however, was uncommonly full of it for more than a fortnight, but as he was perfectly well in every other respect, I never gave him even the usual first dose of saffron tea. Lest some of my readers should be fearful of washing their infants in cold water while this eruption continues, from an idea that it will tend to repel it, I will observe that I never once omitted the washing on that account; but I would wish it to be always understood, that in my method of washing the water is not dashed on in such a manner as to occasion any sudden repulsion of the humour. Indeed I should myself be averse to throwing a quantity of very cold water directly upon the parts where this or any other eruption appears; at the same time I think *washing* with cold water, if it is performed judiciously, is peculiarly beneficial at this time, as the infant's liability to chafe is increased, and its neck and groins will infallibly become sore if it is not done.

Thrush, commonly called the Sore Mouth,

Is far from being so harmless a complaint as that last mentioned; and as I have had but very little experience in it, (as none of my children except the first were ever troubled with it,) I shall not presume to direct others, but give copious extracts from Dr. Underwood, who, from his vast experience in the management of infants, must be peculiarly well qualified to advise and direct, and who has written largely on the subject. After some preliminary observations, he says, "It is among the vulgar errors, however, that the thrush is a very harmless complaint, or is even desirable to a child in the month; for it is said, if it does not then make its appearance, it certainly will at a more advanced age, and will then prove fatal, or, at least, attend patients in their last illness. The fact is, it is a disease of debility, and therefore attacks very old and very young subjects, especially if otherwise weakened. From the above mistake, however, the disorder is often neglected in the beginning, whereby the acidity in the first passages is suffered to increase, which always aggravates the complaint. The thrush indeed is as much a disease as any other complaint which appears in the month, and is connected with most of the foregoing; a proper attention to which, it has been suggested, may very frequently prevent it."

The disorders here alluded to, are costiveness, acidities, wind, &c. and which I think may generally be avoided by putting the babe to the breast as soon as the mother is sufficiently composed to admit of it; to the observance of which salutary practice, and the constant use of cold water, I attribute the happy escape of my children from this distressing complaint. My first child, it is true, had it very bad, but a premature birth, and many other causes, conspired to render him peculiarly delicate, and consequently a fit subject for it. But to proceed with my quotation:

"This disorder is so well known as scarcely to require any description, and generally appears first in the angles of the lips, and then on the tongue and cheeks, in the form of little white specks. These, increasing in number and size, run together more or less, according to the degree of malignity, and form a thin white crust, which at length lines the whole inside of the mouth, from the lips even to the gullet, and is said to extend into the stomach, and through the whole length of the bowels. When the crust falls off, it is frequently succeeded by others of a darker colour; but this is true only of the worst kind of thrush, for there is a milder sort that is spread thinly over the lips and tongue, which returns a great many times, and always lasts for several weeks.

"A principal *remote* cause of this disease seems to be indigestion, whether occasioned by bad milk, or other unwholesome food, or by weakness of the stomach. Perhaps thick victuals, particularly if made too hot or very sweet; also covering the face of the child when it sleeps; or its breathing the confined air of its mother's bed, may be amongst those causes, and ought, therefore, to be avoided. The more immediate cause is the thickness or acrimony of the juices secreted from the glands of the mouth and stomach, producing heat and soreness in these parts. A tea-spoonful of cold water given every morning has been thought a good *preventive;* but keeping the body duly open is certainly better."

With all due deference to the superior skill of this learned writer, I must observe, that I think both ought to be done. I have always made it a practice to put into the mouth of a newborn child a portion of the cold water, before I washed it, for several days; and for the purpose of keeping the bowels open, nature has provided a specific (as before observed) in the mother's breast far preferable to any medicine invented or discovered by art; and therefore a babe ought always to be suffered to suck before the milk *comes.* Every woman knows her bosom to contain a fluid long before her child is born, which cannot properly be called milk, but is undoubtedly designed by an all-wise Creator for a medicine for the infant, and ought to be drawn by the babe before it is mixed with more genuine milk. If this was the universal practice, little aid would be required from art. I observe all the modern writers upon this subject are fond of referring us to the brute creation for examples in the management of our little ones: why, then, are they not consistent; or why direct that an infant must not be put to the breast until the milk comes, as is oftentimes the case. All the young animals which have come within my knowledge (and as I live in the country, I may be presumed to have a chance for observation) suck their mothers almost immediately after they are born. What would become of the tender little lamb, if the shepherd, like some physicians, and *many nurses*, should insist that it should not suck until the third or fourth day after its birth? I believe the woollen manufactory, that great and fundamental support of the British empire, would soon feel the effects of a practice so absurd. Every farmer can tell how absolutely necessary to the health both of the cow and her calf it is, to permit them to remain constantly together the first two or three days after the birth of the calf. To descend still lower in the scale of creation: observe the cat with her numerous family;

how tender she is of her little ones; lying almost constantly with them, and how well they repay her care; how soft, clean and delicate they look: only remove one of these from the mother, and endeavour by every possible care to bring it up, how soon it loses its sleek beautiful appearance; becomes feeble, dejected, and often *dies*, fit emblem of the unhappy little infant debarred by prejudice, or mistaken tenderness, from its own, and only proper nourishment.

> " And can ye then, whilst Nature's voice divine
> " Prescribes your duty, to yourselves confine
> " Your pleased attention? Can ye hope to prove
> " More bliss from selfish joys than social love,
> " Nor deign a mother's best delights to share,
> " Though purchased oft with watchfulness and care."

Perhaps I ought to ask pardon for thus wandering from my subject; but my readers must recollect I do not profess to write systematically, and therefore hope to be forgiven for introducing my remarks when and where they strike me most forcibly. I will now resume my quotations, well pleased to present to those mothers who cannot conveniently obtain the work itself, the fruits of so much real humanity, learning and experience. Dr. Underwood further observes, "The means of cure must be sufficiently obvious, if due attention is paid to the nature and occasion of the complaint. As a general observation, it may be said, that when the thrush attacks robust infants of a costive habit of body, it is easily cured, and indeed requires nothing more than keeping the bowels well open; for which purpose the daily exhibition of castor oil is usually the fittest means. On the other hand, the complaint is attended with some danger in delicate infants whose bowels have been previously weak, and *especially* where the child is *nourished only with the spoon:* much indeed has been said in favour of emetics, especially wine of antimony, as being almost a specific, whatever may be the particular habit of the infant; but I cannot say it has proved so with me; nor can I see any sufficient cause for departing from the more ancient practice in the treatment of this very common complaint.

"I believe, therefore, that where there is no fever, nor any uncommon symptom, testaceous powders are the best and safest remedy; which may be joined with a little magnesia, if the body be costive; or if in the other extreme, and the child is very weakly, two or three grains of the compound powder of contrayerva in its stead. Some such preparation, I mean some absorbent or testaceous remedy, should be administered for three or four days successively, and afterwards something more purgative to carry down the scales as they fall off from the parts. For this purpose rhubarb is generally the best; but when the thrush is violent, of an adust, instead of a white colour; has come on rapidly; and the child is lusty and strong, a grain or two of the powder of scammony, with calomel, may be joined with it; but this must be given with caution. After the purgative, the testaceous powders should be repeated for two or three days as before, till the disorder begins to give way. Afterwards, a tea-spoonful of chamomile tea, or a few drops of the compound tincture of gentian,* well diluted, may be

---

* *Gentian.* Lest, from a similarity in pronunciation, some mistake should arise, it may be proper to notice, that the root here meant is very different from the *ginseng* of our country, both in its taste and pro-

given two or three times a day with advantage; and the bowels be always kept open. On the other hand, when an infant with this bad thrush is weak and delicate, a decoction of the bark with the aromatic confection,* is

---

perties. *Gentian* is described in the Edinburgh Dispensatory, as being of a bright gold colour, and a strong bitter taste; it is found growing wild in some parts of England, and the roots are brought dry from Germany. It is said to lose many of its virtues by exsiccation, and therefore is seldom used as a powder, but forms the capital ingredient in the bitter Wine Tincture and Infusion of the shops; whereas, it is well known that our ginseng is of an agreeable taste, and preserves all its virtues when dry; the state in which it is generally used in common domestic practice.

* *Aromatic Confection.* London Pharmacopœia. Take of zedoary, in coarse powder, saffron, of each half a pound; distilled water, three pints; macerate for twenty-four hours, then press and strain. Reduce the strained liquor by evaporation to a pint and a half, to which add compound powder of crabsclaws, sixteen ounces; cinnamon, nutmegs, each two ounces; cloves, one ounce; smaller cardamom seeds, half an ounce; double refined sugar, two pounds; make a confection.

A more simple mode of preparing this confection is found in the Edinburgh Pharmacopœia, which is said to be equally good:

Take of aromatic powder, three ounces; syrup of

found the best remedy. In regard to applications to the part, it is necessary to observe, that as they have little to do in curing the complaint, it will be improper to have recourse to them very early.

"If, therefore, the inside of the cheeks and tongue are covered with thick sloughs, or foulness, it may be convenient to clean the mouth two or three times a day; but otherwise it will be improper till the complaint is past the height, the sloughs disposed to fall off, and the parts underneath inclined to heal;

---

orange peel boiled to the consistence of honey, six ounces. Mix them by rubbing them well together so as to form an electuary. See Edinburgh Dispensatory, pages 548, 549. This aromatic powder is thus prepared. Take of cinnamon, lesser cardamom seeds, and ginger, each two ounces; reduce them together into a powder, to be kept in a well stopped phial. See Edinburgh Dispensatory, page 523.

This powder is an agreeable, hot, spicy medicine; and as such may be taken in cold phlegmatic habits, and decayed constitutions, for warming the stomach, promoting digestion, and strengthening the tone of the viscera. The dose is from ten grains to a scruple and upwards.

which never takes place until the secretions in the first passages are become bland and mild.

" Proper applications will then have their use, not only by keeping the mouth clean, but by constricting and healing the raw and tender apertures of the little vessels of the cheeks and tongue.

" Of these preparations, a variety have been in use, in the form of lotions and gargles, which from the earliest times, have all been of an astringent nature. Borax is certainly one of the best, and may be mixed up with sugar, in the proportion of one part of the former to seven of the latter: a pinch of this put upon the child's tongue will be licked to all parts of the mouth; but made into a paste with common honey, (about two scruples or a drachm to an ounce,) it will hang about the mouth better than in a powder. Either of these, however, may be, at this period, made use of as often as shall be necessary, to keep the parts clean; which they will effectually do without putting the infant to pain by being forcibly rubbed on. I must own I have frequently been distressed at seeing nurses rub the mouth of a little infant with a rag mop, as they term it, till they have made it bleed; and this operation they will often repeat half a dozen times a day."

I perfectly agree with this humane writer, in censuring this cruel practice, and thank him for making known a method so much more consonant to the feelings of humanity. I have been more copious in my extracts upon this subject, because I know the error of regarding this complaint as rather salutary than otherwise, exists in our country; and as I have every reason to think my own child was injured for want of due information on the subject, I would wish to warn others from so prejudicial a mistake, that they may, by proper and timely attention, either prevent the disease entirely, or render it far less injurious.

I can likewise inform my readers, that our country boasts, among a vast variety of vegetable productions, a plant generally known by the name of dragon root, or wild turnip, that is an excellent remedy in this complaint, and for the canker in all its forms. It is used in the same manner Dr. Underwood prescribes borax. I am not scientific enough to describe technically the virtues of this root; but I know that when fresh it resembles a common English turnip in its appearance, is of a smart pungent taste, so much so, as to render it almost intolerable; but after it is perfectly dry, it loses most of its pungency, and becomes extremely hard, so that it must be grated when used. In this state, if taken in large doses, it will operate as an emetic, and for that reason is found efficacious when infants are much oppressed from a cold, if given repeatedly in small potions, by loosening the cough, and gently exciting them to throw up the phlegm. It is also known to be very good for the colic, either for very old or very young patients. I frequently give a small quantity grated into water, and sweetened a little, to my infants, when they appear afflicted with pains in the bowels, and generally with great success.

Snuffles.

THIS complaint, though very troublesome, is not frequently attended with any hazard to the child: and for all cases of the common snuffles, I know of nothing better than anointing the ridge of the nose with a little sweet oil, and at the same time rubbing some of the same oil on the soles of the feet, and warming them some time at the fire. This will generally procure instantaneous relief: but when this could not with convenience be done, I have found milking a little breast milk up the nose produce the desired effect: it will generally make the infant sneeze, and by that means clear out the head, or by otherwise softening the hard matter which usually occasions the complaint, remove the difficulty.

But if the difficulty of breathing through the nose should frequently return, and at length be attended with a copious discharge of purulent matter, resembling that from a bile, and accompanied with evident debility, without any other precise complaint, there will be reason to apprehend the *morbid snuffles* have occurred, and the best medical advice ought instantly to be procured; as this, so far from being a slight or common complaint, is a very dangerous and dreadful disease.

But the better to enable parents to distinguish it, that, when it does occur, it may be properly and seasonably attended to, and that the fond mother should be spared any unnecessary alarm, I will again avail myself of Dr. Underwood's authority, and insert his description of the symptoms and general management of the disorder, lest no medical assistance could be with convenience procured, as I find, even in London, many physicians were unacquainted with this disease.

"This disease, like all other disorders, is much more violent in some instances than others. In all a peculiar attention must be paid to the bowels, especially that they be kept more than commonly open; and to attend to the nurse's diet if the infant be suckled.

"But it may be necessary to be rather more explicit on this disorder, than on many others that may be considered as above the management of ordinary readers; because the complaint being as yet but little known, and more dangerous than would be apprehended, it might not otherwise be sufficiently distinguished from the effects of a cold, until it would be too late to attend to it with effect.

"It was first noticed in 1790; and the most formidable symptom found to be the difficulty of breathing through the nose; though this is not constant, and when free from it, children *appear* to be in no danger: but the difficulty at other times is so great as to require an attendant to watch the child, sleeping and waking, in order to open the mouth as often as may be requisite. A singular purple streak is likewise noticed at the verge of the eyelids, and which may be considered as a precise mark of the disease. A general fulness is also observable about the throat and neck externally, taking place soon after the commencement of the complaint; which may be properly dated from the appearance of the purulent discharge from the nose: though it has been remarked that this symptom, although one of the most formidable, may be entirely wanting.

"When the above symptoms have continued for some time, according to the strength of the patient, and degree of the disease, children become pale and languid; at this time also the glands of the throat become swelled, and of a dark red colour, with ash-coloured specks upon them, and in some there are extensive ulcerations. The infants gradually decline in their strength, and have a particular catch in respiration. They are unable to suck, though not universally; they swallow with difficulty whatever is given to them in a spoon; and *die in convulsions,* or with all the marks of great debility, though not on any particular day of the disease.

"The true source of this disorder appears to be a defluxion and inflammation over all that extent of membrane that lines the posterior nostrils and contiguous parts. Hence, the copious secretion of purulent matter irritates the windpipe, and produces that spasm, and croaking noise, with recurring sense of suffocation, so uniformly observed in this disease. By descending into the stomach and bowels, it disorders those parts, and if not very soon properly treated, induces such general disease as greatly debilitates, and at an uncertain, but generally at an early period, carries off the little patient in the manner already described.

" From this account of the disorder, a regard to the state of the bowels is the manifest indication, which must be more attended to than in almost any other disease; since the keeping them very open, so as to prevent the lodgment of the matter falling into them, is the grand means of cure. To this end, one or more tea-spoonsful of castor oil should be given every day, so as to procure four or five motions daily. If the child should be weakened by these means, some cordial medicine should be interposed; or should this prove insufficient to support the infant, the purgative must be somewhat abated: but it is remarkable, that even weak infants endure purging better under this complaint than perhaps any other, unless it be the tooth-fever.

"It is necessary to add, that though this complaint had never till very lately been met with after the month, I have seen one instance of it in an infant of a quarter old; who was nevertheless thought, I know not how justly, to have had some slight symptoms of it in the month."

I have thus given my readers such a description of this distressing disease, with the best method of cure, as I think will enable them to guard against its more pernicious effects. And I have been induced to do this, from having, formerly, been a great sufferer for want of such information. I have a lovely little girl, who I suspect had it. She was attacked with it when only a week old, and the discharge, with all its distressing symptoms, continued for several weeks; with sometimes a day or two of intermission. Unfortunately, the medical gentlemen I applied to were unacquainted with the disease (and at that time I never had heard of it); therefore, although their applications succeeded in curing the complaint in the head, yet, as little attention was paid to the bowels, the child languished along until three months old, when, after being uncommonly unwell for several days, she was seized with convulsions, and had twenty-three dreadful fits in the course of one week; these naturally called for every aid, and were at length relieved by calomel, which brought away stools so green as to be almost black: from which it was evident the cause was then in her bowels. I immediately recollected her early complaint, and was convinced that was the prime cause of her long ill state of health, and finally of the fits; although I knew not its appropriate name. After the operation of the calomel, however, she slowly recovered, and I had the supreme felicity of being assured by the physician who attended her, that my unremitted care and attentions, both before and after the last dreadful attack, were a great means of enabling her to struggle through her complicated complaints!

Say, ye fair votaries of dissipation, who, amid the gay delirium of the rout, the ball, the concert, and the play, drown all recollection of your maternal duties, when did either of your favourite amusements yield a sensation to be compared with the blissful idea of having in the least degree contributed towards saving the life of a beloved child? O, believe me, you widely deviate from the paths of exquisite enjoyment. I do not ask, I do not expect, every mother to devote herself as I have done to her family; I know the laws of society will not admit of it; but I would have every mother *taste*, at least, of the pure unadulterated cup of joy prepared for her by her beneficent Creator, and presented only by her *children*. It is from them, in their sweet endearing caresses, their unsophisticated manners, and unfeigned affection, that genuine happiness is to be found, enhanced by the consciousness of having done our duty to them.

> " Ah yet, ye fair, shall come that happier day
> " When love maternal shall assert her sway,
> " And crowning every joy of married life,
> " Join the fond mother to the faithful wife;
> " When every female heart her rule shall own,
> " From the straw cottage to the splendid throne;
> " Nor e'er, for aught that fortune can bestow,
> " A mother's sacred privilege forego."

Wind in the Stomach and Bowels.

WIND is well known to occasion many alarming appearances in very young infants: indeed, from the birth until four or five months old, they are more or less troubled with it, and sometimes longer; but with proper care, I fancy little danger need be apprehended from it. Dr. Underwood attributes the more violent effects, such as spasms, convulsions, &c. to indigestion, improper food, and especially costiveness; but I know that infants may be very much afflicted with wind, who never took any other food than their mothers' milk, and were in apparent good health in their bowels in every other respect; nevertheless, I have not the least doubt that such infants, if they should be improperly fed, would suffer infinitely more; and think every mother ought to be very careful about her diet, when she finds her infant peculiarly subject to this complaint. I have often observed my children to suffer greatly, after I had incautiously indulged myself in eating apples, or other flatulent food. I then make it a practice to correct my milk, by drinking an infusion of some of the carminative herbs, or seeds; such as catmint, pennyroyal, or caraway. The essence of peppermint is very good, as the effect it has is almost instantaneous. The infant should always have something given it, likewise, whenever it appears distressed with wind in any way whatever. The most common symptoms are rolling about the eyes while asleep, starting and crying out suddenly, also crying violently, and drawing up the legs, as is the case in all pains of the bowels, from whatever cause they may proceed. I have been in the habit of using various little remedies, such as dragon root, the roots of the peony, ginseng, and sweet flag.

and essences and distilled waters from all the aromatic seeds, among which I give the preference to anise and caraway. The roots may be used in the form of powders by grating a little into water, warming and sweetening it to render it agreeable. The essences must be used with caution, or they will be apt to quackle very young infants; one or two drops will be sufficient at first in a little warm water, and if there should be occasion to use them often, the child will gradually bear, and indeed require more. The distilled water is preferable, when it can be procured; a great spoonful of this may be given, with the addition of a little sugar, and if it should prove too strong (which may be known by the child's catching its breath after swallowing a little of it) it may be diluted with common water. Dr. Hugh Smith observes, that infants are often affected with a complaint similar to what we call the heart-burn, and recommends giving them a little magnesia as the best remedy. I do not pretend to judgment enough either to confirm or refute this elegant writer; but I have frequently found a tea-spoonful of magnesia, given in a little caraway or mint water, or even common water, quiet an infant to sleep, and appear to render it perfectly easy when every thing else failed. The best way of giving it is to take the quantity you wish to give, and put it in a large spoon, braid it very fine with your finger, so as to be sure there are no lumps in it, then fill the spoon with whatever you have prepared to give it in, mix it, and cause your babe to swallow it as quick as possible, as the magnesia loses much of its absorbent quality by being wet; and a small dose given in this way, will have a better effect than double the quantity forced down, after standing wet in a cup until every particle is perfectly saturated with the liquid. I have always used large quantities of this innocent and excellent medicine among my children, and never knew it fail of having a good effect in acidities in the stomach and bowels, and I believe, if it was constantly used in small quantities every day, it would tend greatly to prevent watery gripes, and many other distressing complaints incident to infants, provided they are not killed with kindness, by having their tender stomachs daily crowded with pap and other preparations altogether unnatural and unnecessary. Dr. H. Smith, in his Letters to Married Women, inveighs with more than usual energy against the absurd practice of feeding such young infants with pap, and it has already been seen with what conclusive arguments Dr. Underwood combats the custom. I sincerely hope the united efforts of these, and other gentlemen of the faculty, will have their due weight with every judicious mother, and prompt her to banish all such pernicious preparations from her nursery. Milk is the only proper substitute for the breast, and I verily believe if infants were never suffered to take any other, many of the disorders always so distressing, and often fatal to them, would be avoided.

The elixir paregoric I have always esteemed a harmless and salutary anodyne for infants; and have found it very serviceable in sudden colds, hoarseness, or coughs, and peevishness, which is ever occasioned by pain. I have been cautioned against using it, from an idea that infants accustomed to take it would not sleep without: but I can truly say I never found the least difficulty in discontinuing it whenever I pleased. It is undoubtedly very wrong to give it to a healthy child every night, as is the custom with some, merely to favour the attendants by quieting it to sleep: and it is certainly best *never* to give infants medicine if it is possible to avoid it; yet of two evils I would always choose the least, and it is cruel to let a sweet little creature endure hours of pain, until a strong constitution triumphs over the complaint, or a weakly one sinks under it, merely from an apprehension that the patient *may* be injured by taking medicine. It should be the care of every intelligent mother to improve her judgment by consulting the most approved medical books on the treatment of children; but more especially by observation and attention to their constitutions and complaints, and thus qualify themselves to judge when nature really requires assistance, and how to administer it with propriety, in all *common complaints;* for I must here beg leave to enforce upon my readers one *solemn* precaution. If your infants are really ill, so that their complaints will not readily yield to the common palliatives, or the often greater efficacy of good nursing, let me entreat you not to delay calling in professional aid until your children are too far gone to admit of relief. Thousands of helpless little innocents suffer greatly from the too prevalent opinion (especially among the lower classes of society) that a physician cannot tell what to do for such young children. In the hope that such parents may be convinced by sound reasoning, I will insert what a very able writer says upon the subject. Speaking of the idea we are now considering, and the consequent want of timely attention to the complaints of infants, he says, " But I may venture to assert, that although infants can give no account of their complaints in the manner of adults, their diseases are all plainly and sufficiently marked by the countenance, the age, the manifest symptoms, and the faithful account given by the parent, or an intelligent nurse. This I am so confident of, that I never feel more at my ease when prescribing for any disorders than those of infants, and never succeed with more uniformity, or more agreeably to the opinion I may have formed of the seat and nature of the disease. Limited as is human knowledge, there are yet certain principles and great outlines as well in physic as in other sciences, with which men of experience are acquainted, that will generally lead them safely between the dangerous extremes of doing too little or too much; and will carry them successfully where persons who want those advantages cannot venture to follow them.—Let me ask, then, is it education, is it observation and long experience, that can qualify a person for the superintendence of infants, or the treatment of their complaints? Surely all these fall eminently to the share of regular practitioners, to the utter exclusion of illiterate nurses and empirics." I trust no judicious parent will dispute arguments so conclusive. But there are those who believe all medical aid superfluous; that if persons are to die they will die, and that to endeavour to save life by human means is a species of profanation. Is, then, the benign art of healing the invention of man? Did man by his own wisdom discover the various properties of the innumerable plants which compose the materia medica of nature? Even allowing this; did man *give* to those plants their *virtues?* Did he impregnate the bowels of the earth, and the "vasty deep," with minerals, fossils, and the various testaceous substances, so wonderfully adapted to mitigate the diseases incident to fallen man? Surely not; and no one will presume to doubt the *Infinite Wisdom* that did. Is it not equally presumptuous to say all this was done for no end; or that *He* who teaches the brute creation to cull from his immense stores the simples adapted to their diseases, did not likewise place in the heart of his favoured creature Man, a more acute discernment, joined to a judgment little less than divine.

Retention of the Urine.

As this is a complaint which sometimes causes great distress, it ought to be attended to immediately. An infusion of the leaves and root of the common mallows, I have sometimes found have the desired effect, or parsley roots steeped very strong, and a little of the tea given sweetened with honey is very good; but for very young infants I never found any thing preferable to a tea made of pompion or pumpkin seeds; this never failed to remove the complaint whenever I have had occasion to use it among my children. Dr. Buchan observes, that "a warm bath of milk and water, or a little oil gently rubbed on the belly, will in most cases prove efficacious." If after all these methods have been tried, the retention should continue, skilful advice should be had, as the impediment may be occasioned by some defect which ought to be immediately attended to.

Sore Ears and Eyes.

THESE often troublesome and disgusting complaints will generally be entirely avoided, by washing an infant constantly with cold water, as directed in the beginning of this chapter. The first of them, however, will sometimes occur, notwithstanding every precaution, and I think when it is only a slight discharge, unattended with an eruption, I should be careful of using any violent applications to check it; as it may be a salutary exertion of nature, and may prevent more fatal complaints: but great care should be taken to prevent the excoriation from extending itself, by washing the part every morning, or oftener, if necessary, with warm milk and water, or a weak suds of Castile soap, and carefully placing behind the ear a piece of scorched linen. If this should fail, a little plaster of Turner's cerate may be applied; or a weak solution of sugar of lead may be used instead of the other washes. But I have of late found a very little opodeldoc, dissolved in warm water the most efficacious application I ever tried in this complaint; and it will generally prove effectual, if persevered in a sufficient length of time. Every mother and nurse ought to be informed, that one great reason why many applications and medicines are condemned as ineffectual, is, because the use of them is too hastily suspended, before sufficient time is allowed for their due operation.

As the eyes are a more delicate organ, I will give my readers Dr. Buchan's own words upon the subject; especially as none of my children have ever been affected with the least complaint in that part.

" Sore eyes are in general occasioned by the neglect of washing the infant's head with cold water from the birth. Where that method is practised, this complaint seldom occurs: though it may sometimes happen by exposing it soon after birth to a strong light, or placing it too near the fire. In both cases, the most simple applications are the safest; and frequent washing with milk and water, or rose water, will in general remove all the disagreeable effects of this disorder."

Vomiting.

There are many opinions with respect to infants throwing up their milk. Physicians generally suppose it a symptom of too great acidity in the stomach; but for my part, when it is done without any appearance of nausea, I regard it rather as an indication of strength than otherwise; and as a kindly exertion of nature to free herself from any superfluous quantity received into the stomach. I am inclined to think it not a disease, from several reasons: in the first place, it is generally observed to be the most thriving children who do it, and those who are nourished from a very full breast of milk. It is also a fact, that infants most generally throw up their milk while in the act of playing and springing with every appearance of glee; which would not be the case, if they felt sick. Indeed, this has always been the criterion by which I have always been accustomed to judge if the vomiting proceeded from illness, or was only the effect of repletion. If my babe at the moment hangs its head, looks uncommonly pale, or by affecting moans shows evident indisposition, I immediately conclude its stomach out of order, and treat the complaint accordingly; but otherwise I always regard it rather as an indication of health and strength than of disease. However, whenever, from the symptoms above related, I have had reason to think the vomiting proceeded from acidity in the stomach, I have ever found magnesia an effectual remedy; or if that should fail, it is probable the complaint proceeds from something offensive in the first passage, and a gentle emetic of ipecacuanha may be given: three grains, or half a tea-spoonful of the ipecacuanha is generally sufficient for children of this age; and if that should fail to remove the complaint, a weak infusion of senna and manna may be exhibited, until it produces a gentle operation; a table spoonful may be given every two hours until it operates. After this the magnesia, or any of the testaceous powders may be repeated a few times, and will rarely fail of having the desired effect.

Convulsions.

ALTHOUGH this cannot be termed a slight or common complaint, yet as no disorder that ever attacked my family gave me such acute distress, or so totally overpowered my faculties, I cannot resist the desire of giving some account of it, together with the most approved method of treatment; lest some fond mother, while her heart throbs with agony for a beloved child, should find it impossible to obtain medical aid immediately, and may take up my book, with the eager hope of finding the directions she requires. I recollect with what anxiety I sought for information, when my child was so unexpectedly seized with these fits, and cannot think any further apology necessary for transcribing copiously from Dr. Underwood, relative to the usual causes and remedies; leaving the reader to consult that learned author for more particular information as to the *various kinds of convulsions,* if she should be so unfortunate as to have occasion so to do.

" If it may be accounted a fair rule of judging from the result of my own experience, both in hospital and private practice, convulsions ought not to be reckoned amongst the most frequent disorders, and are certainly far from the most fatal to infants; perhaps as many as nineteen cases out of twenty having their appropriate and almost certain remedies.

" Such original cause may be a rash improperly repelled, but the source of fits is much oftener in the gums, in the time of teething; or in the first passages, where some undigested matter, or merely pent up wind, irritates the coats of the intestines, and produces irregular motions throughout the whole nervous system. Instances of this kind have been related of children, who, during the first months, have had frequent attacks of violent convulsions, which have disappeared entirely upon the prohibition of meal pap. Indeed, too much caution can scarcely be given on this head, thick victuals being a more frequent occasion of convulsions in young children than is commonly imagined. Any offensive load, whether from too great a quantity or bad quality of the food, by occasioning a faulty secretion, must act like a poison; and that the convulsions are owing to this cause, may often be known by the complaints that have preceded them, such as loathing, costiveness, purging, pale countenance, large belly, and disturbed sleep. Every young infant is, however, more or less predisposed to this complaint; and the disposition continues throughout childhood, in a proportion to the tender age and delicacy of the habit. The younger and more irritable, therefore, an infant may be, it will be so much the more liable to convulsions, especially from any considerable disturbance in the first passages, as was mentioned before, particularly from the bad quality, or over thickness, of the breast milk or other food, and from frights of the wet nurse. Of this I remember a remarkable instance in a patient of my own, in whose house a visitor suddenly dropped down dead. The mother of the child, which was six months old, was exceedingly alarmed; but her attention being for a moment called off by its crying, she incautiously put it to her breast. In an hour afterwards the infant was seized with a fit, and lay either convulsed or drowsy, without so much as taking the breast, for the space of six and thirty hours; though it was at length happily recovered, as infants in such case generally may.

" Among the various causes of convulsions (though equally the occasion of many other complaints) may be mentioned that of foul air, and want of cleanliness in the dress and other accommodations of infants ; against which the lower class of people only need to be cautioned.

" Of a like kind, probably, was a curious case I met with very lately in an infant of only a fortnight old, who was suddenly seized with convulsions without any manifest cause. They had gradually increased for three days when I was called to visit it, and notwithstanding a fair trial given to almost every medicine I had ever made use of for fits, they continued for six weeks, and for the last three became almost constant, so that except during the short sleeps the infant got, it was rarely five minutes together out of a fit. The last week I attended, all medicines were given up; but the fits continued the same, and the infant, reduced to a very emaciated state, was now expected to expire from one hour to another. As a last resource, the child was taken to the country, where, to the surprise of every one, the fits left it, the infant having only two through the whole of the next day, and none afterwards. The sudden recovery can only be attributed, I imagine, to change of air.

" The cure of convulsions of whatever kind will consist principally in removing the exciting causes, which must therefore be inquired into. If from improper food and indigestion, a gentle emetic should be given; if the irritation be in the bowels, whatever will carry down their acrid contents will cure the convulsions, if administered in time; and we ought generally to begin with a clyster.

If the stools appear very foul after common purges, (in which case there will frequently be some difficulty of breathing,) a few grains of the powder of scammony with calomel, may be given with great propriety. But, if the disposition to convulsions continues after the bowels have been properly cleansed, and no new irritation of them may be apprehended, the proper remedies for spasm should be administered, such as tincture of soot, or of castor, spirit of hartshorn, rectified oil of amber, or oil of rue, which, though an obsolete medicine, is an excellent one: but to begin with any of these, as is sometimes done, is as hazardous as empirical. Rubbing the back bone, palms of the hand, and soles of the feet, with oil of amber, or water of ammonia, has likewise had a good effect, as well as frictions over the whole body, which from consent of parts seems to afford more benefit than might be imagined."

I have thus given a brief detail of the common sources from whence this distressing disorder may be expected to arise, and likewise the best remedies; and were I not fearful of swelling my volume far beyond the limits I have proposed, I could with pleasure extend my extracts from this valuable work: I must, however, insert one passage more, for the consolation of every mother who may be alarmed for the life of her child while labouring under this complaint.

" A few more words may be necessary, especially as they hold out much comfort in regard to this alarming complaint. For though indeed all convulsion fits are in their appearance extremely shocking, yet, under proper treatment, it has been remarked they are much less frequently fatal than is commonly imagined, however often they may recur; and for my own part I do not recollect more than three infants dying in convulsions during the last five years, though I have attended several who have had more than twenty fits in a day."

When I reflect upon the comfort such an assurance, from such authority, would have given me when my darling child was afflicted by them, I feel a sincere hope that in giving it a place in this little volume, I may chance to alleviate the distress of many a fond mother.

Fever, from taking Cold.

This kind of fever may very easily be distinguished from any other, by its being preceded and attended with the usual symptoms of a cold; and I mention it here, because I think by proper and timely care, and good nursing, one of the most dangerous disorders incident to infants, an inflammation on the lungs, may be avoided: to this end, when an infant is in the least degree feverish when afflicted with a cold, especially when attended by a cough, the feet and legs should be bathed in warm water, and drafts applied to the feet; and for young children, garlic drafts* are to

---

* *Garlic Drafts.* To make these drafts, simmer the cloves of garlic in olive oil or hog's lard, then cut some brown papers about the size of a dollar, dip them, and apply them to the soles of the feet, binding them on with proper bandages. These drafts are very excellent for young children, because they are very easy to the feet, are easily renewed by dipping the papers anew, and are very powerful in their effects upon the system. Dr. Sydenham assures us "that among all the substances which occasion a derivation or revulsion from the head,

be preferred, both for their peculiar virtues, and being easy to the feet: this done, half a tea-spoonful of the oxymel of squills may be given in a little hyssop tea, sweetened with honey ; and if the infant is relaxed in its bowels, or subject to griping, six or ten drops (according to the age of the child) of elixir paregoric may be added: the mother or nurse should drink, when going to bed, a bowl of catmint tea, or any other cooling herb she may prefer. If the child should not be apparently better the next morning, the bathing, drafts and squills may be repeated: this, with great care to keep it from the cold, and that all its clothes are perfectly dry, will generally alleviate the complaint; but should the fever continue, the breathing become difficult, with a flushed cheek, an inflammation on the lungs is to be feared, and immediate recourse should be had to some approved physician ; but I

---

none operates more powerfully than garlic applied to the soles of the feet." Hence the good effect in febrile affections, especially in this complaint. I have, however, found them equally efficacious for older children, when afflicted with worm complaints.

have often found the above method of treatment, persevered in for two or three days, procure relief in very severe colds. The syrup of squills I would particularly recommend, in almost every affection occasioned by taking cold: where that cannot be had with convenience, a gentle emetic of ipecacuanha should be given; three grains, as mentioned before, is generally sufficient for such young infants; but if that should not operate sufficiently to give relief, the dose may be increased to four or five without danger: as, if you apprehend the operation to be too violent, it may be easily checked by a few drops of paregoric; but this seldom happens with this emetic, which has, besides, this peculiar quality, that if it does not operate as an emetic it will as a purgative, and often have the desired effect without puking the infant, which I think should be done with caution while they are so young. Nevertheless, in this complaint, it appears absolutely necessary, as the little creatures have not discretion to expectorate in the usual manner, and therefore, unless relieved in some other way, become very much oppressed with phlegm: they also swallow large quantities with their milk, which renders it indigestible, and thus induces general disease; therefore it will be proper to keep the body duly open; for which purpose a weak infusion of senna and manna, given gradually until it operates, will have a good effect, or half a tea-spoonful of magnesia may be given twice a day; this I confess is a favourite medicine with me for very young children. One thing more I would observe, as the measles and some other eruptive diseases begin with every appearance of a cold, it will be proper to give a child so affected, saffron tea several times, as that will tend to throw out any latent disorder of that kind, if requisite, or by its stomachic and exhilirating qualities prove otherwise serviceable. I know not why the learned colleges in Europe have seen fit to invalidate the virtues of this very excellent plant. It is *undoubtedly* one of the best we have; and indeed whatever indisposition attacks my children, my first step is to give a dose of this tea, and I am pretty sure if there is any peccant humour lurking in the blood, it will then make its appearance on the surface.

It may not be improper to mention here, that whenever *honey* is used medicinally, it should previously be boiled and skimmed, as otherwise it is very apt to occasion acute pains in the bowels, and to some constitutions is almost a poison. I would therefore suggest the propriety of always boiling it before it is put up for medicinal purposes, as we are frequently called to use it in haste, when it may be impossible to attend to this precaution.

On cutting the Tongue.

This is an operation so simple and so easily executed, that no mother need to hesitate a moment about performing it herself, as I have done for several of my children with perfect safety and success; by taking a pair of very sharp scissors, and holding them between her fingers very near the points, so as to preclude the possibility of cutting more than the very outward edge of the string that confines the tongue, and thus avoid all danger of cutting too far, or wounding any of the veins beneath the tongue; from which it is said infants have sometimes bled to death. Another danger arising from this operation is said to be *suffocation*, from the child's swallowing the point of its tongue, and which is owing to cutting *too much* of the string or bridle; but I can truly say, that although there may be danger of one or both these dreadful consequences, yet I verily believe any judicious mother may perform the operation without the least apprehension, provided she feels sufficient resolution: otherwise she had better employ some professional gentleman to do it. My babe, who is now in arms, had his tongue tied to the very end, so that whenever he cried or attempted to lift his tongue, it was drawn into the form of a heart. As soon as I was able to attend to him, I seized an opportunity when he was asleep on my lap, and, gently placing the fingers of my left hand under the tongue, I took a pair of nice scissors, and, in the manner above directed, with ease severed so much of the string as allowed him to suck with freedom, and the babe never awoke or appeared to feel it in the least: but I soon found the operation was not complete enough to permit the tongue to move as it ought to do; and when he was two months old, fearful lest it might cause some impediment in his speech, I cut the string a little more, and although the child was then awake, he never showed the least uneasiness by which I could suppose it caused him any pain, but smiled the whole time. His tongue bled a very little, and ever since has appeared perfectly free.

SECTION V.

On the great Utility of alternate Exercise and Rest, with Observations on the pernicious Practice of taking Infants out of Bed during the Night when in Health.

> Say who is he, so debonair
> With active limbs, and sportive air,
> With step elastic, bounding, there
>   In frolic gambols sporting?
> 'Tis *Exercise;* and by his side
> See *Health,* his constant blooming bride,
> In all the flush of rosy pride
>   Delighted with his courting
>
> And now upon the violet bed
> He droops fatigued his weary head,
> In gayest dreams illusive led,
>   His daily toil renewing.
> Refreshed by sleep, at early dawn
> Again he frolics o'er the lawn,
> And gathers roses to adorn
>   The bride he's ever wooing.

AFTER all that has been said concerning the management of infants in sickness or in health, perhaps nothing will tend more either to prevent the one or insure the other than *exercise.* The first week of their existence new born infants may be permitted to sleep as much as they incline to, but even then they should be frequently moved, and gently rubbed with a warm hand to excite them to stretch; and as soon as they show a disposition to open their eyes, they should be encouraged to do so by gently tossing in the arms, moving from side to side, or in any other way inducing them to look about. As they grow older, the exercise should be increased, and when the season will permit, and the weather is fair, they should be carried abroad every morning, and permitted to breathe the fresh air for an hour. In this way their health will be greatly benefited, and their minds will appear to open much earlier, than if they were continually hushed to sleep by artificial means: they will generally after their morning's walk or ride fall asleep, and awake, after resting an hour or two, with renovated strength, and even their mental faculties expanded. Thus they will soon acquire such a proportion of knowledge as will no longer submit to confinement, but by a restlessness arising from an inherent love of variety, oblige their attendants to carry them from place to place; and as soon as they begin to notice persons or things, they should be constantly talked to, and their attention drawn to familiar objects by frequent repetition. This will excite them to spring forward themselves, which will give a more effectual start to the blood, than hours of moderate movement, such as infants usually obtain from their attendants. Thus weakly and delicate infants will

> " Acquire a vigour and elastic spring
> " To which they were not born"—
> ARMSTRONG.

and the more robust have a good constitution firmly established.

Mothers and nurses will eventually lessen their own fatigue by thus permitting their infant charge to have sufficient exercise; for true it is

> — " Repose by small fatigue
> " Is earned"—
> ARMSTRONG.

and children will usually sleep sweetly during the night when they are not permitted to sleep too much in the day, and are duly wearied with the exercise they have taken. Thus the mother's rest will be unbroken, and she will awake in the morning refreshed and invigorated; her milk will be infinitely better, her health and strength be confirmed, and she will feel able to arise and attend to her maternal duties with delight.

> " Then loveliest, when her babe in native charms
> " Hangs on her breast, or dances in her arms."

To this end, I must be permitted here to censure the too prevalent custom of taking infants out of bed in the night, a practice which cannot be too strictly guarded against. It is astonishing with what facility the little creatures will learn bad habits; or with what ease they may be made to acquire good ones. I have frequently been vexed to hear parents complain of their children, and aver that they *would not* lie in bed, but cry to be taken up and see the candle; for I always suspect the parents only are in fault. With a mistaken spirit of indulgence, they will not permit the dear little creatures to complain in the least, but the whole house must be disturbed to appease them: or from a more reprehensible impatience of fatigue, many mothers will summon their attendants if the child is in the least degree restless; without reflecting that those who are wearied with continual labour through the day ought to be suffered to sleep quietly during the night, unless something of great importance forbids it. The infant is taken up, and shortly, from the powerful force of custom, acquires a habit of waking exactly at such an hour, and this probably for many months, to the great disturbance of both parents and attendants. How infinitely better were it to endure the small inconvenience of attending a very young infant for a few nights in the bed, until it should learn to lie still, than by thus causing them to be taken up upon every slight pretence, confirm a habit productive of incalculable fatigue, and equally destructive of comfort and health.

With all my numerous family I never had an infant taken out of bed during the night, after the first month; nor then, except for the purpose of obtaining dry clothes, (after which I always take them immediately to bed again,) except they were ill; and I verily believe they never would require it if they were not injudiciously managed at first.

Thus, my fair friends, I have endeavoured to state what I believe to be the best method of nursing and managing infants from the birth until they are four months old, and in the pleasing hope that if you have adopted my advice your babes are thriving, fair, and lovely, I will now proceed and assist you all in my power through the difficult period of teething. And may that *Almighty Being,* who knows the purity of my motives, give efficacy to my feeble efforts for the preservation of this lovely and interesting portion of society.

CHAPTER II.

SECTION I.

On Teething, and the Management of Infants during the often painful and critical Period of Dentition.

"I've often heard my Grandame say,
"When she was young that roguish Fay
"Would spirit brawling brats away,
"And in the cradle where they lay
"Would leave their elvish changelings.

"Now watch with care the techy babe,
"And learn the spell which Grandame said
"Would charm the Sprites. A *Mother's* arms
"Are potent 'gainst all fairy charms;
"And in their hallowed bounds will keep
"The babe from Oberon's deceit."

WE are now to suppose our infant charge arrived at that age when its sweet endearing smiles and innocent caresses begin to interest every beholder. How infinitely interesting then must they be to a mother who has watched with impatient fondness the first dawn of its rational faculties, eager to catch the earliest indication of our noble and exalted nature! How amply is she now repaid for the many hours of fatigue and anxiety spent in nursing its earlier infancy! This may be imagined by the effect produced on the foster nurse. How frequently do we hear it observed that she scarcely perceives any difference in her affection for her nursling and her own offspring.

> " Leaps his young heart with undissembled bliss
> " At the fond look, soft smile, or gentle kiss;
> " Whilst by his lips the milky orbs are prest
> " The soft affections spring within his breast,
> " Till the pleased hireling owns the tender claim
> " And to a mother's office joins *the name*."

Ah, how is she to be pitied who is *obliged* thus to yield her sacred right to the earliest affections of her babe—and still more so that mother who *voluntarily* sacrifices such *heartfelt bliss,* for the empty pageantry of fashionable dissipation! Now every day, nay, every hour, some new charm is disclosed, some fresh emanation of mind unfolded, and some novel and fascinating gesture displayed. Let those ladies who seek variety in their pleasures, and yet banish their babes from their bosoms, be persuaded for once to try the talisman of infant blandishment, and they will acknowledge they have at length found that variety which chases the ennui of life. And here also we find our beneficent Creator has graciously blended our pleasures with our cares; for now our infants call for particular attention; it being absolutely necessary for their health, if not their very existence, that they should be faithfully nursed and constantly exercised and amused for several months of this portion of their lives, and the better to ensure those advantages, their heavenly *Father* has clothed them with such enchanting loveliness as none but brutes in human form could possibly resist: hence every one is induced to notice them; they are frequently handed from one to another, each trying by every possible means to excite a smile, or other token of regard, and thus they acquire new ideas, and receive the exercise best adapted to promote their health. Now, too, the little creatures begin to drink more deeply of the bitter cup of mortal infirmity, as this is the age when they usually show the first indications of pain from the irritation of their gums, and often appear to suffer greatly even before there is any appearance of the teeth, either from the gums swelling or becoming inflamed, probably owing to the teeth shooting through the bones. Rubbing the gums at this time is said to be of service, " as it not only somewhat appeases pain, as adults sometimes experience in the common toothach, but it also forwards the growth of the teeth by drawing more nourishment to them, as well as assists their irruption, by pressing the gum and nervous membrane firmly against their points." The application of honey, or the syrup of white poppies, to the gums at this time is likewise recommended.

It has long been thought by many, almost indispensable to furnish infants with the coral and bells, both as an amusement and assistant in the irruption of their teeth, but I have entirely thrown aside mine, being fully convinced that infants generally prefer to bite something that will yield more to the pressure than coral: and however they be at first attracted by the jingling sound of the bells, they soon grow weary of them, disgusted rather than amused by the monotonous sound and glittering appearance, and will throw them aside for a less gaudy toy, especially if they are in pain. I have been led to this conclusion from observing, that whenever, from a wish to amuse them when fretful, I have jingled the bells before their eyes, they would avert their faces, and, sinking upon my bosom, seem to entreat me to desist: and while I reflected upon the distress we feel in after life, when tortured with pain at the teasing recurrence of any noise whatever, it appeared altogether unnatural to attempt amusing a sweet little sufferer by a means that would almost distract a much older patient. Besides, it should ever be remembered that the infant mind, eager for information, can receive no new ideas from the jingling of bells or the shrill toned whistle, and that every purpose of amusement is much better effected by talking to them, and new ideas constantly conveyed: thus I said to my babe to day, George where is **Rover**? at the same time pointing to a favourite spaniel which lay upon the carpet: the dog advanced, and the child sprang forward delighted; and now when he is asked where is Rover? he immediately looks around to find him; thus he has acquired an idea productive of constant pleasure. On reading this passage to my little circle, Amelia ran to her brother Edward, clapping her hands and exclaiming, Oh, Oh, mamma has put Rover in her book! This was followed by a lecture to my audience upon the nature of printing and vending books, and the pleasure and profit of reading them; when my eldest son, who thinks himself very profound in Greek and Latin, with a dash of the pedant natural to his age, gravely observed to his father, "If mamma would but study Greek, and write her book in that language, Rover might become immortalized like Ulysses' dog in the Odyssey." Thus we endeavour to connect amusement with profit, in the various grades of infant and juvenile life. But to return to my subject: The very best assistant in this way to the irruption of the teeth is a cork. Take a corkscrew and worm it into a new cork of a proper size to be admitted with ease into the mouth, and you have a plaything both useful and pleasing to the child; the soft and spongy nature of the cork is exactly suited to the tender state of the gums, and is unattended by the danger inseparable from permitting such young infants to chew a crust of bread, which is often recommended; but they too frequently get off large pieces, which might be productive of fatal consequences unless great attention was paid, and this cannot always be obtained from ordinary attendants: and the ivory or ebony head of the common corkscrew I believe equally good as the coral, when a more polished substance is required; and if of gold or silver, they are still better. I have observed an infant set several minutes at one time and bite the cork, with evident tokens of pleasure, while his little hands were busily employed playing with the corkscrew. It is my opinion that a due attention to air, exercise and amusement, is the chief requisite to ensure comparatively easy dentition; but great care must be taken to *keep* infants in health at this time, for although teething cannot, perhaps, properly be termed a disease, it is often attended by, or productive of many disorders; such as long continued constipations, convulsions and fevers, or violent diarrhœa, and consequent weakness of body: various kinds of rash likewise frequently appear at this time, and may generally be esteemed salutary. But although thus menaced on all sides by various complaints, infants who have been properly managed from the birth, and nourished entirely by milk, will generally triumph over them all, and most commonly escape them entirely; therefore, I will notice such complaints as sometimes occur in the healthiest children, and unless very much neglected, scarcely deserve the name of diseases. We find almost every child will be either very costive or greatly the reverse at this period, and it should be the mother's peculiar care, to watch these symptoms, and afford the necessary aid in due time; in either case no alarm need be felt while the child appears in good spirits, has a good appetite, and does not by unusual fretfulness, or any other *marked* symptom, evince certain indisposition: and here again the all-wise hand of the great Creator is displayed, for not more true are the indications of the magnetic needle, than the aspects of the infant countenance; and as the skilful mariner, by noting the one, conducts his vessel safely to her destined port, so may the judicious mother, by observing the other, judge accurately of her infant's health. I never feel in the least anxious about my children while their eyes are bright and lively, their faces dressed in smiles, and they show a *constant* disposition to play; (by which I would infer that the partial ebullitions excited by endeavours to amuse them do not reach my meaning;) but when they look pale and dejected, their eyes dull and heavy, seldom irradiated by a smile, it is beyond doubt that they are ill, and require some little medicine to assist " oppressed nature in her arduous task." If the child is strong and robust, it will be most inclined to feverish complaints, attended by constipation, in which case I have always found magnesia answer a very good purpose, especially if the child is affected with acidity in the stomach and bowels, which will generally be the case. The magnesia may be given in doses of a tea-spoonful to infants from four to six and seven months, in a little peppermint, or caraway water, sweetened with manna, before going to bed, and repeated in the morning, if it has not the desired effect. Magnesia, however, will not always operate as a purgative, and when this happens, and the complaint proves obstinate, the best medicine I ever tried is syrup of elder berries: a tablespoonful will be sufficient for an infant of six months or under, and after that the dose may be increased to two table-spoonsful without danger. I have known this effectually remove a disposition to constipation, which would not yield to other purgatives, and leave the children in perfect health for many months. Rhubarb should be avoided, as its astringency will but aggravate the complaint. Dr. Underwood recommends a medicine which some ladies may wish to try, especially as it is highly recommended both as a laxative and cordial, and may be of service whether the child is too costive or greatly the reverse. "Take of rhubarb fifteen grains; half a drachm of magnesia; sweet fennel and dill waters, of each six drachms; half an ounce of syrup of roses, and ten or fifteen drops of the compound spirit of ammonia; of this, one, two, or three teaspoonsful, according to the age of the infant, may be given two or three times a day."—

Weakly infants, on the other hand, will generally be most inclined to diarrhœa during the progress of dentition; and it is well known that great caution should be used not to check it too soon, as infants always cut their teeth easiest when their bowels continue very open. Dr. Underwood, when treating upon this subject, says, "It has been observed that a purging is beneficial; and it may be proper to add that it is surprising how considerable it may be on this occasion, and how very bad the stools, for several weeks together, and the child happily struggle through; though at another time an equal degree of purging, with such bad stools, and constant fever, would prove infallibly fatal. The purging is therefore not only to be cautiously treated, according to the directions already given under that article, but is generally rather to be increased than suppressed." Therefore, it will be best to do little else than give a little magnesia, or any of the testaceous powders, in catmint or mint water, every day, so as to counteract gently the disposition to acidity, and warm the bowels, provided the babe is otherwise in health; but if the disorder should continue too long, and violent, so as greatly to weaken the child, some further attention will be required; and then the medicine before recommended (and which is said to keep some time) will be of great service, and should be repeated occasionally as may be found requisite. When this complaint has continued some time, infants so afflicted will frequently appear pale and languid, especially in very warm weather. In which case Dr. Underwood recommends a cordial medicine to be given on the intermediate days, or in the evening, after the operation of the medicine: " Take of the aromatic confection, a scruple; spearmint water, an ounce and a half; dill-seed water, half an ounce; syrup of tolu or saffron, a drachm; compound spirit of ammonia, ten drops; a tea spoonful may be given for a dose. As cordials are frequently mentioned, the above may serve as a general guide, and may be made more or less warm by a greater or less quantity of the aromatic confection or spirit of ammonia." If these gentle means fail, the following may be tried.

" In the early part of this disease, the active purges are the most proper, such as castor-oil, senna, and sometimes calomel; or if the fever be considerable, an infusion of burnt sponge and senna in boiling water, a preparation equally adapted to the fever and this kind of purging. This should consist of two parts of senna leaves (by weight) to one of burnt sponge, made of such a strength that the bowels may bear one or more table-spoonsful, two or three times a day. The infusion, as soon as it becomes cold, should be strained through filtering paper."

While infants are breeding teeth, their evacuations will often assume a jelly-like appearance, frequently streaked with blood, which causes the anxious mother much alarm, lest the dysentery has occurred; but I believe that dreadful disease is generally distinguished by very appropriate symptoms, being always attended with loss of appetite, fever, and extreme pain: the discharges also, though very frequent, are in very small quantities; the very reverse of the diarrhœa usually attendant on dentition, which is seldom accompanied with fever, and infants will usually preserve a good appetite, although the disease should prove obstinate and troublesome. Nothing therefore will be necessary, should such instances occur, but occasionally to repeat the medicines above recommended, and to pay every possible attention to their diet, not suffering their little stomachs to be loaded with improper food. If the mother has milk enough, the child will require little else, except in occasional absences from her, when milk new from the cow is the best substitute, if it can be procured; if not, something as nearly resembling it as possible should be prepared. A very excellent beverage both for food and medicine, in cases of obstinate relax, may be prepared by boiling a handful of dry flour tied up in a cloth very close, several hours, until it becomes perfectly hard and dry; it may then be grated with a common bread grater, and a table-spoonful stirred into half a pint of boiling milk, so as to make it like thin panada; a small piece of cinnamon should be added to the milk, and when it is boiled sufficiently, it may be sweetened with a little loaf sugar, or not, as is most agreeable to the child. Infants are usually fond of this food, and may be permitted to eat a few spoonsful several times a day as a medicine, or a tea-cupful instead of other food when necessary. I have frequently found this simple diet have a better effect in disorders of the bowels than any other medicine, after proper evacuations had been made. The flour when thus boiled will keep many months, and may be prepared occasionally, as a variety in the food of children of even two or three years old, when afflicted with bowel complaints of this kind; and is excellent in the real dysentery. But, after all, let me repeat, do not suffer this complaint to cause any unnecessary alarm, although often very troublesome, unless your infants appear otherwise ill, nor induce you to administer astringent medicines without good advice, as many infants, I fear, lose their lives from having this salutary effort of nature injudiciously counteracted. Gentle anodynes given at bedtime, I think of infinite service, as they do not operate as a check except for a few hours, procuring both the nurse and the child necessary rest, and by that means the infant acquires a degree of strength to bear the pains and evils of the day. They tend likewise, more than any other medicine, to allay the irritation, which is often the principal cause of the disorder; and I have been assured by experienced physicians, that physic will usually have a better effect, if preceded or followed by them, than it otherwise would. It is frequently asked, especially by young mothers, which teeth are cut first? and in what order do they advance? As it may be gratifying to some to have these questions fully answered, I will state the usual progress of dentition, agreeably to the observations I have made among my little tribe.

Children generally begin to show evident signs of pain and irritation in their gums about the third and fourth months, and seldom cut all their teeth until nearly two years old, and sometimes even later. The first teeth commonly appear in the lower jaw, the two directly front are usually cut first, then two immediately over them, then one on each side in the upper jaw are seen to advance nearly together, then one on each side the two first teeth in the under jaw; these eight are in general all that appear in the first year; but there *are instances* when twelve or fourteen are cut in that time. The next teeth which make their appearance are two large double teeth, one on each side in the under jaw, then the correspondent ones above, then the eye teeth as they are called, and so on in regular succession. But it will sometimes happen otherwise, and the teeth will advance very irregularly, which may be considered as pretty good evidence that the dentition is difficult and painful; which is often the result of improper management, or unhealthy parents: hence, probably, has arisen the vulgar opinion, that children who cut their side teeth first never live to grow up, for it is a melancholy fact that weakly children too frequently die during this critical period, and often before any teeth appear; a striking instance of which is recorded by Dr. Hugh Smith, to enforce the great efficacy of lancing the gums.

" A poor woman in the neighbourhood some time since brought her child to me: he was apparently a stout fine boy, and then about nine months old. She desired my advice for an eruption the child had all over his body, which she called scurvy; but I found nothing more than some pimples, proceeding from the improper quality of its food: and in fact, notwithstanding the chubby appearance of the boy, (which in reality was nothing more than bloated fat,) he was actually of a very weakly frame, as appears by the sequel. Near or quite six months afterwards, the same woman came to beg the favour of me to look at her child again, who she said was dying. I saw an infant worn away to a mere skeleton; and upon inquiry found it to be the same chubby fat boy I had seen before. It lay panting for breath, and had taken little or no nourishment for twenty-four hours. Upon examining the little patient, there was not a tooth appeared: the cause of the disease therefore was immediately evident to me; but I told her it was too late to be of service, for I found the child could not recover. However, to satisfy the mother, I advised lancing the gums. To the astonishment of every one, sixteen large teeth were cut out; but the gums being very much hardened for want of this operation, it was with no small difficulty performed. The immediate relief the child received surprised them all still more: from a convulsive state that he before lay in he instantly recovered, took notice of every body in the room, and, during the time I staid, eagerly devoured a considerable quantity of nourishment. The grateful parent thanked me a thousand times, and reflected upon herself for delaying to apply to me before. But alas! I foresaw it was only a temporary relief, his strength being utterly exhausted. I left her without giving the least hopes of his recovery; and the next morning the child died. A reflection upon this case, I take for granted, is entirely needless. It is evident had the teeth been cut in due time, this fatal accident would not have happened."

Every mother must feel the force of this story; may it prompt the most vigilant attention! I sincerely hope the safe and salutary practice of lancing the gums will soon become universal, as I am confident it will save many lovely little sufferers much extreme pain, and most of these alarming complaints. But as I know many very tender mothers are really fearful of having the operation performed by a physician, I must beg them to adopt a mode I have always practised, and which answers a very good purpose, although perhaps not quite so effectual as the regular method. I take a very keen razor, and wrap the whole blade in a fine handkerchief, leaving only the extreme point uncovered, (to prevent all danger of wounding the mouth,) and with that make an incision in those gums which appear to cause the pain, always making it a point to feel the razor grate against the tooth, and then I am pretty sure it will advance without difficulty. I have often done this when the gums were very much swelled and inflamed, and the child in such distress as to require every exertion to keep it tolerably quiet: in half an hour afterwards, the whole edge of the teeth, where the incision was made, have been visible, and in the course of a few hours the inflammation has subsided, and the infant appeared surprisingly relieved. I always perform this simple operation as the infants lie asleep in my lap, nor do I recollect a single instance of their awaking from it. It generally occasions a slight bleeding, which is of itself serviceable, if we may credit the assurances of many eminent physicians who have written upon the subject. Dr. Underwood has favoured us with many excellent directions and opinions upon this subject, which I will transcribe for the benefit of those who cannot conveniently purchase so large a work, or may not have time or inclination to peruse it. " When it is found necessary to lance the gums, (which is ever at least a *safe* operation) it should always be done *effectually*, with a proper gum lancet, and not with a needle, a thin six-pence, or such like instrument, which will not sufficiently divide the gum, nor the strong membrane that covers the teeth. The lancet should always be carried quite down to the teeth, and even be drawn across the double teeth. It is certain that this little operation gives scarcely any pain, and the relief is at the same time often so considerable, that the child immediately manifests it by squeezing the jaws, and grinding them together forcibly; which proves they are not very sensible. The most painful part of teething, and that in which children are most exposed to convulsions, is usually from the teeth cutting through the nervous membrane that covers the jaw immediately under the gums. This, I apprehend, in difficult dentition, is often not cut through, but is forced up before the teeth, when they are even in sight, under the thin gum: hence it is, that cutting through the gums is so very often useful, and takes off fever and convulsions, which severe symptoms could not arise merely from teeth piercing through the gum, which, it has been said, is not a very sensible part. At other times, the pain and fever seem to arise from almost the very first shooting of the teeth within the jaw, and then they will very often not appear for some weeks after the gums have been lanced; and parents are apt to conclude the lancing has been unnecessary, if not improper. *I am, however, convinced from experience, that this little operation, though not in the general esteem it ought to be, is often inexpressibly useful, and appears to have saved many lives, after the most dangerous symptoms had taken place, and every other means of cure made use of.* The mere *bleeding from the gums* is capable of affording some relief, as it is frequently found to do in adult persons distressed with the toothach. And I cannot here forbear expressing my surprise at the fears some people entertain of lancing the gums, and their delaying it so long, if not altogether rejecting it, though no evil can possibly arise from the operation. On the other hand, its advantages are so great, that whenever convulsions take place about the usual period of teething, recourse ought always to be had to it after an unsuccessful use of other means, though by an examination of the gums there may be no certain evidence of the convulsions being owing to such cause; the irritation from teething, it has been remarked, sometimes taking place in a very early stage of the business. At any rate, (it is repeated) the operation can do no harm even at any period; and should the shooting of teeth be only an aggravation of the true cause of the disease, lancing the gums must be attended with advantage. But should teething be the proper and sole cause, it is evident how fruitless any other means of relief must frequently be; for should convulsions, for instance, take place from a thorn run into the finger, or toe, the proper indication of cure, by an immediate extraction of the thorn, is evident, and the futility of other means must be equally obvious." Much more is said by this learned and experienced author on this subject, but I shall content myself with extracting one passage more, as it appears to touch a point where I myself am peculiarly sensible, from having seen a beloved child greatly afflicted, and I naturally feel a particular desire to guard every mother from the agonizing sight of an infant in convulsions! After many other arguments in favour of lancing the gums, he says, " Purging, fever, and *even convulsions,* will sometimes arise from only one point of a large tooth offending the nervous membrane that covers it, and being nearer the surface than the other points, the lancet may sometimes not completely divide the membrane that lies over the rest, (or it is afterwards healed,) and this part not being injured by the tooth, the symptoms subside on having divided that portion of the membrane that was inflamed. But in a little time another point of the same tooth is found to irritate this sensible part, and calls for the like assistance, which again removes all the complaints. I have seen the like good effect from it, when children have been cutting a number of teeth in succession, *and have bred them all with convulsions;* nothing having relieved or prevented these terrible symptoms but *lancing the gums,* which has removed them every time it has been done, one or more teeth appearing a day or two after each operation." Convulsions are particularly to be dreaded at this period, as they are said often to attack children very suddenly who appear to enjoy fine health, (excepting the pain from their gums,) and thus a mother may be taken by surprise, and obliged to witness the agonies of a darling child, when totally unprepared for so shocking an event. Therefore, I sincerely hope, what has been said upon this subject will have its due weight with my fair readers, and prompt them to conquer any latent fears they may entertain, while thus assured by gentlemen of undoubted skill, humanity and experience, that no danger can possibly attend the operation, but every advantage may reasonably be expected from it. Surely it is absurd to pretend to such extreme sensibility as to be unable to see an infant's gums lanced, whilst we live daily spectators of the most excruciating pain which it will almost instantly relieve. Thus do we see the pampered daughters of pride and luxury avoiding with horror and dismay the abode of poverty and sickness, lest a sight of the wretched inhabitants should agonize their too susceptible hearts; when their presence and friendship might relieve the keenest pang of merit in distress, and their superfluous wealth, properly employed, cause the "widow's heart to sing for joy!"

Air and exercise are of the utmost importance at this time. A variety of good effects will arise from permitting the little creatures to be carried abroad almost constantly. Change of place and new objects will amuse them, and we all know the efficacy of amusement in the common toothach. By air and exercise likewise, general health is induced, which will ensure safe, and comparatively easy dentition. And I verily believe, that infants who are nursed by their mothers, managed from the birth as directed in the preceding pages, and permitted to breathe the fresh air, with proper exercise every day, will seldom meet any difficulty, or be seriously affected with any of the complaints which have been here noticed, during this often critical and dangerous period of their infancy, but may thus be carried forward until nine months old in health and safety, which is the best time, in my opinion, to wean them.

SECTION II.

Observations relative to teaching Infants the right Use of their Hands.

> " *Now*, when his little hands from bondage free,
> " Restless expand in new-born liberty,
> " You teach the Child, with reprehension light,
> " In preference to the *left* to use the *right*."
>
> Roscoe.

The anxiety many parents discover, lest their children should be left-handed, may excuse my devoting a page or two of this book, in endeavouring to combat an idea pretty generally entertained, that it is necessary to watch an infant when it first begins to use its hands and direct it

> " In preference to the left to use the right."

It is my decided opinion, that if a child is *left-handed*, it is a natural defect which it will be impossible ever entirely to overcome; and although the infant might, as it advanced in life, be taught to use the right hand so well as greatly to obviate the inconvenience and awkward appearance arising from it, yet the propensity would always predominate, while a child which has not this natural defect, will never acquire it after birth, and therefore all anxiety upon the subject is superfluous. That this is as much an insurmountable defect as any other natural deformity, may be inferred from the rarity of its occurrence, and that, generally, whenever it does occur, it is observed to be hereditary, and often all the children of the same family will inherit it as a legacy from their parents. Therefore, although I would by no means wish to deter mothers or attendants from using every proper means to counteract a defect so disagreeable in appearance, and inconvenient in its consequences, where they actually discover it to exist, yet I must believe no inattention whatever on their part can ever be censured as the cause of such a propensity in children who have it not born with them. If want of care and attention could produce this effect, we should probably much oftener discover this characteristic mark of the ancient Benjamites among the labouring part of the community, who, from the necessity of constant occupation, seldom have time or inclination to attend to these little niceties in their children, and, provided they can procure them " food to eat and raiment to put on, therewith are content;" and probably seldom think of the circumstance until the child has decided the point by evincing beyond dispute which hand it prefers to use: and yet I fancy the defect does not occur more frequently among that class than in the more polished circles.

SECTION III.

On the best Time and Method of setting Infants on their Feet.

" See the plumed Parent teach her callow care
" With outstretched wing to scale the ambient air,
" Tempts with maternal note the rude essay,
" And lures the infant bird from spray to spray:
" Lo ! on the ground the unfledged flutterer lies,
" The meadow echoes with its infant cries;
" With eddying wing the parent stands confest,
" And all the Mother flutters in her breast;
" Till by degrees the timorous pupil knows
" To beat the air and perch the trembling boughs;
" With pinion strong to mount the azure sky,
" And fill the groves with native minstrelsy."

It is universally known that infants, *if well*, will show a disposition to get upon their feet very young, often as soon as the fifth or sixth month: indeed, if a child is strong and healthy, it will appear evidently pleased to stand on its feet before it is six weeks old, and even earlier, and undoubtedly this natural propensity

" To walk erect, and raise the eye to Heaven,"

should be indulged as soon as the little creatures acquire strength to hold themselves upright. But it is a certain fact, that it is not always the most thriving children that go alone the youngest. Slender, delicate infants, if they enjoy good health, will often walk very young; while a heavy child, although equally healthy, will not venture until twelve or fourteen months old. So that we may fairly judge that this is no certain criterion by which to estimate an infant's health. At any rate, they should never be enticed to go by any artificial means a moment sooner than they incline. Their natural propensity to imitation will incite them to evince a desire to get upon the floor as soon as they are capable of the least comprehension, and to walk as soon as they are able; therefore, they should be permitted to sit or creep about a carpet as long, and as much, as they please, care being taken not to leave them sitting in one posture too long; and even until their affecting moans grow too painful to be any longer endured, as is too often the case in the middling and lower classes of society: whereas, I verily believe that even those mothers who are compelled to work for their subsistence, would eventually find their account in attending more than they usually do to their infants during the first year at least, or until they are firmly on their feet, and can exercise themselves sufficiently; for I greatly fear many an unfortunate little creature becomes deformed and rickety, from no other cause than want of exercise and attention, who would, if properly attended, have contributed in a few years to the support and comfort of its parents. Children who are permitted to creep about the room as much as they please, will usually prove more elegant in their forms, and strong in their constitutions, than those who are forced upon their feet too early; therefore, their attendants should be instructed to hold them up occasionally by a chair or other convenient place, suffering them to sit down whenever they please, so as to avoid the possibility of distortion, from keeping too long in one posture, at the same time that they learn by degrees the use of their feet, and they will soon show their tractability by stepping round the chair; and by a thousand enchanting looks and gestures, assure us that they are sensible they have learnt something new. After this, they may be led about the room, the attendants standing behind them and holding both hands. I have frequently trembled to see a heavy chubby infant swinging by one arm, and often twitched up at the imminent hazard of dislocating the limb; a cruel and pernicious custom, which can never be adopted but by very thoughtless or very unfeeling attendants. Thus the little adventurers may be led on from step to step, until they acquire discretion to venture alone, which they will undoubtedly do as soon as their limbs have gained sufficient strength and elasticity, from an intuitive desire of imitating those around them, and perhaps a still stronger propensity to wander from place to place, which they will soon perceive they cannot readily do unless they can walk. I have often observed that they will go alone when they have something given them to carry, long before they will venture without, which evinces that it is frequently the *apprehension* of falling only that deters them from walking; therefore they will sometimes gradually lose their fears by being often excited to walk with some object which will wholly occupy their attention; for instance, by standing at a short distance, and calling them to take a toy or cake that you hold in your hand, and, as they advance, stepping gently and almost imperceptibly back, so as to decoy them on: this, however, must be done dexterously, without permitting the children to discover the deceit, or they will rarely be deceived a second time. Great care also should be taken to prevent their falling during these early essays; as they will frequently refuse to attempt walking alone for some weeks, after having received a contusion on the head from an unlucky fall backwards, although previously it appeared probable they would

> Trip nimbly round the gay parterre
> With bounding step, and frolic air,

in far less time. For this, and other reasons above enumerated, it may be best to suffer them to tumble about a carpet, or lead them whenever they show a great desire to walk, until they voluntarily venture alone: this will afford almost equal relief to the attendants, and prevent all danger of accident, or distortion, from falling, or confining them too long in one posture. Happily, those pernicious inventions the go-cart, standing stool and walking stool, are rapidly growing obsolete, and nature begins to assert her sway in that as in many other particulars of infant management; and **I** sincerely hope they will ere long be consigned to complete oblivion, together with the *scull caps, forehead cloths, swaddling bands* and *stays*, in which our great grandmammas used to imprison their hapless offspring. **I** have heard my grandmother relate, that one of her sons walked down cellar in a walking stool and almost killed himself.

Hence we see it will not do for us to draw analogous conclusions from the brute creation, in this article of infant management at least; for, designed by nature to seek their own food, and take care of themselves, they are formed by the hand of infinite Wisdom with athletic limbs and instinctive perceptions suited to their necessities, while the helpless little infant is consigned to our care, a weak tender little being, formed to arouse the softest and the finest feelings of our nature, "a bundle of tender vessels," calling for constant care and attention, or it must inevitably perish; and such it remains in a degree for many months, gradually acquiring strength as its mental perceptions unfold themselves, rendering it in some measure aware of the dangers that surround it. Hence we perceive the first passion children discover is *fear;* awakened, doubtless, for wise purposes, by their divine protector. As their strength increases their fears subside, until at length we see them advance by little and little, feeling their way, till finally

> " They spring exulting, like the bounding roe;"

which, that they may be enabled to do, it will be necessary, as early as their health and the seasons will permit, to let them feel their feet unconfined by clothes. Infants' clothes should be shortened as soon as they incline to stand upon their feet, or show a desire to get upon the floor, unless the weather should prove inclement at that time; if so, it will be best to defer the innovation to a more propitious season. On the other hand, if the infant will arrive at a proper age (which I think may be fixed at five or six months) at a season when the winter begins to advance, it may be better to shorten them a month or two earlier, as no danger need be apprehended from the change, provided the weather is warm, and infants will walk the younger for feeling their feet at perfect liberty. Some ladies insist, in compliance with the fashion of their vicinity, that the poor little creatures must continue enveloped in an exuberant length of muslin and other articles of dress until twelve months old, when probably they would have ran about rejoicing in less time but for that incumbrance. Others again never put long clothes on their infants at all, and we see their little tender feet exposed to all weathers from the birth. Both these extremes are to be deprecated; as it conduces to the health and comfort of a very young child, to keep its feet wrapt from the cold, not less than it contributes to the welfare of one of six months old, to use them as much as it will.

A mother's cares, however, do not cease when her infants are firmly on their feet. Then, like the unfledged bird, they are always overstepping their bounds, or incautiously venturing too far. She feels far more secure while her babe only creeps about, and she can close the door upon its excursions. When once they feel themselves capable of walking like other people, they are impatient of confinement, and wish to roam at large; few attendants are to be trusted with them; too often the child is permitted to wander, while the servant is otherwise engaged, until some precipice or pitfall arrests its feeble steps. But where shall we place the boundary of a mother's fears, or how prescribe for their relief? It is found *only* in a sincere and humble reliance upon that omniscient Being, who suffers not a "sparrow to fall to the ground unnoticed," And here she may *rest* secure that the pious effusions of a mother's heart, committing her children to his protection, shall never be in vain.

CHAPTER III.

SECTION I.

Directions as to the best Manner and Time of weaning Infants, and the Diet best adapted to promote their Health, after they are weaned.

> " Since there's no help, come let us kiss and part;
> " Nay, I have done, you get no more from me;
> " And I am glad, yea, glad with all my heart,
> " That thus so clearly I myself can free."
>
> DRAYTON.

THIS is perhaps one of the severest trials a mother is called to endure; and no one can possibly conceive the pang she feels, when compelled to relinquish the sweet office of nurse to her babe, but those who have themselves experienced its fascinations. What sensation can equal the rapture of that moment,

" When the fond mother, bending o'er his charms,
" Claps her fair nursling in delighted arms;
" Throws the thin kerchief from her neck of snow,
" And half unveils the pearly orbs below;
" With sparkling eye the blameless plunderer owns
" Her soft endearments and endearing tones,
" Seeks the salubrious fount with opening lips,
" Spreads his inquiring hands, and smiles and sips."
DARWIN.

Nevertheless, the dreaded hour will come, when she must forego all these soft emotions, and therefore it is best for every mother to arm herself with resolution, and determine, when the proper time arrives, not to delay the task until her babe shall increase in knowledge, and by a thousand endearing blandishments render it infinitely more painful. Reflection only adds to the difficulties instead of removing them; and it may be said with truth in this, as in a more important sense,

" She who deliberates is lost"—

her maternal tenderness will conjure up a thousand alarms for her infant's health, which I verily believe are altogether ideal, although I must confess I have felt their soul-subduing effects again and again: but we shall always find this, like most of the ills and perplexities of life,

—" Shrink from the eye of firm resolve,"

and become more or less formidable, in proportion to the pusillanimity or firmness with which we meet them. Let us then set about the business with good courage and perseverance, and we shall find the performance of this task far less distressing than the contemplation of it.

There has been much learning and many arguments displayed by different writers, both for and against the necessity of habituating infants to take other food than the breast previous to this event. Dr. Hugh Smith advocates the practice; Dr. Wallis also is decidedly on that side. Dr. Buchan, speaking on this subject, says, in favour of feeding them after the fourth month: " This will ease the mother, will accustom the child by degrees to take food, and will render the *weaning* both less difficult and less dangerous. All great and sudden transitions are to be avoided in nursing. For this purpose, the food of children ought not only to be simple, but to resemble as much as possible the properties of milk: indeed, milk itself should make a principal part of their food, not only before they are weaned, but for a *long time after.*" On the other hand, Drs. Underwood and Thompson esteem it a matter of no material consequence, whether done or left undone. Among these clashing opinions of the learned, if my fair readers will accept of the fruits of my experience, it will be found rather on the side of the last-mentioned gentlemen, as I have frequently observed that some children, who appear to crave every thing they see others eat, and would, if permitted, eagerly receive various kinds of food during the earlier months, as they advance towards the usual time of weaning, grow more and more attached to the breast, and finally refuse all other nourishment before they are twelve months old, and thus render it necessary to break them at once from all connection with their mother, when the period arrives that they must be weaned: and others, who never appeared to wish for any food whatever, except that which nature provided for them, and could not be enticed to drink even milk without great difficulty, when, owing to the absence of their mother, they are compelled by imperious hunger to take something; and others again, who were always equally happy, whether they were permitted to suck or fed with the spoon; and yet all these children weaned equally well. Therefore, I cannot give up the belief, that it is nowise material; but nevertheless, I would always *wish* (in conformity to the idea advanced by **Dr.** Buchan, "that all sudden transitions should be avoided") to have an infant pleased with its milk, and somewhat habituated to eating it, either with or without bread, before the weaning commences; but it rarely happens that a child arrives at the age of nine, or especially *twelve months* old, without being more or less accustomed to other food than its mother's milk; their propensity to imitation would render it almost impossible to keep them from partaking in the meals of their attendants in some degree, after they arrive at an age to make known their desires, so that little apprehension need be felt on the score of a too sudden transition. The greatest difficulty arises from the danger of their being overfed.

Meats of all kinds should be *positively forbidden*, except in broths and jellies; those may be occasionally allowed, when a change of diet is esteemed necessary, but the longer children are fed upon milk the better: plain bread and milk is the most proper food for infants when first weaned, and for many months afterwards, if they are weaned within the first year, which should always be done, if possible; and I believe it will be conceded by physicians, that children fed in this simple manner, for *several years* will enjoy better health, generally, and when attacked with any of the purulent disorders, stand a better chance for their lives, and suffer far less, than those who are fed profusely from a luxurious table every day. Milk may be prepared in various ways to give variety to their food: custards are both innocent and nutritious: rice boiled until perfectly soft in water, and then milk added to it and again boiled, and then rendered palatable with a little cinnamon and sugar, is generally pleasing to infants, and is calculated to prevent a diarrhœa, which is said frequently to attack children upon this change in their diet: but I have never found it have that effect on mine, and I am apt to think when it does happen, it is often the effect of overloading their stomachs with improper food. They may be rendered very happy without the aid of cakes, sweetmeats, or pastry; but lest I should be thought too rigid, I will take the liberty to recommend a simple cake, which is not only innocent, but often beneficial to them. Take a quart of treacle, add to it half a pint of good sweet cream, three eggs, two tea-spoonsful of pearlash, and two ounces of ginger, and stir in fine flour until it becomes of the usual consistence of poundcake; it may then be baked in pans of any form you fancy, and the children be allowed to have a small piece several times a day, so as not to overload the stomach, as the great art of feeding young children consists altogether in providing them proper food, in such quantities that they may be frequently hungry, and as frequently have their appetites indulged. Whenever a child leaves part of its cake or bread and butter, it is pretty good evidence that the little creature is *ill,* or *improperly fed,* which amounts to nearly the same thing. In order to make children enjoy their good things they should always be *rarities:* if they are permitted to have cakes and sweetmeats in profusion every day, they will soon lose their charm, and give no more delight than a simple piece of bread would, to a child differently treated. The cake above mentioned, will be very light, and the ingredients are all such as will conduce to the infant's health, whether it be inclined to too long constipation, or the contrary extreme. This may appear doubtful to many of my readers, but I have *proved it,* by experience, to be equally beneficial in both cases, and a little reflection upon the nature of the ingredients will convince the judicious mother of the *probability, at least,* of the fact. This cake, then, and milk in the various forms in which it may be prepared, with sometimes an addition of broth and jellies, will be amply sufficient both for the health and gratification of infants, until nature provides them teeth to chew more substantial diet; and till this is the case, they should, on no account, be fed with animal food. I have seen the most baneful effects produced from indulging an infant too freely in this way, even after it had a number of teeth. Children of this age have not discretion to chew their meat properly, and they eagerly suck it down in a state wholly unfit for digestion, especially in the tender stomach of an infant. One of my children came very near losing his life from this cause. He was a remarkably healthy boy, and always showed a great inclination to eat whatever he saw others eat; but as this was inadmissible in my opinion, I always restricted his diet agreeably to the above system, and forbid all his attendants indulging him with any other without my express permission: one evening, however, he was suddenly seized with vomiting, threw up all his supper, and from every appearance, I suspected he had eaten something improper: the servant, however, who had attended him the past day, denied all knowledge of the fact, and I attributing his illness to some other cause, sent for a physician: when he arrived, the child had fallen asleep, and little could be done, ignorant as we were of the cause of the complaint: the child had a restless night, looked miserably in the morning, and every thing he attempted to swallow was instantly returned. I then gave him a gentle emetic, but being young and inexperienced, I was fearful of dabbling in medicine, consequently did not give enough to produce much effect: it gave him some relief, however, and he continued dosing the chief of the day, and towards night revived a little, and took a light supper, but evidently with no great appetite: shortly after the vomiting returned with great violence, and he threw up more than I should suppose his little stomach could possibly contain; his countenance grew ghastly, his strength failed, and, greatly alarmed, I again summoned the physician, who prescribed rhubarb and ipecacuanha, leaving four powders to be given night and morning until it relieved him: when he had taken only two of those powders, he threw up large pieces of *veal,* which he had sucked down almost three days before, and which were now of a *dark green dingy colour, and extremely fetid.* The servant was then compelled to acknowledge she had, in compliance with the wishes of the child, fed him with the veal, and alarmed at the consequences, feared to acknowledge it. I have been thus particular in relating this occurrence, in hopes to impress upon *mothers,* and all who have the care, of infants, a sense of the fatal effects which may arise from an injudicious indulgence of their appetites: and also caution them to examine their servants very strictly, should any such symptoms occur, that proper means may be used in due season for their relief. Had the girl who attended my child candidly acknowledged her imprudence, the physician, when first called, would have known how to proceed, and the babe escaped much distress. Had he been out at nurse, or neglected at this time, it is altogether probable he would have fallen a sacrifice to this mistaken indulgence. This child was eighteen months old, and had been weaned nine months.

With respect to the expediency of sending an infant from its mother to be weaned, no general rule can be given; as many children will mourn more for *her* than for the breast; especially if she has been in the habit of attending upon them principally herself, or permitted them to be almost constantly with her. It may be best, therefore, to regulate our conduct in this particular entirely by the disposition of the child; and as some will be very obedient and contented, if suffered to remain with their mother, and others cannot be pacified unless kept entirely from her, their feelings only ought to be consulted when about to lose their earliest joy. If an infant is peculiarly attached to its mother, independent of her character as nurse, it seems cruel to deprive it of all comfort at once; and no mother can possibly hesitate what line of conduct to pursue, when her child thus evinces beyond dispute that it is *her*, and not the food, he mourns for. No indulgence, no attendance whatever, can compensate to a child of this description, the loss of maternal endearments.

> " Ah what avails the cradle's damask roof
> " The eider bolster, and embroidered woof?
> " Oft hears the gilded couch unpity'd plains,
> " and many a tear the tassel'd cushion stains!
> " *No voice so sweet attunes his cares to rest,*
> " *So soft no pillow as his mother's breast!*
> " Thus charmed to sweet repose, when twilight hours
> " Shed their soft influence on celestial bowers ;
> " The cherub *Innocence,* with smile divine,
> " Shuts his white wings, and sleeps on *Beauty's* shrine."
>
> DARWIN.

If we thus consult their feelings, and attend to their diet and amusements, infants will seldom droop or seem in the least unwell from weaning; but they will frequently appear thoughtful, and lose their vivacity for a day or two, and no wonder; for who, in more advanced life, would bear to be deprived of their dearest enjoyments, and not evince far greater dejection and impatience. The remedy is self-evident; the babe must be amused by every possible means, and not suffered to ruminate upon its sorrows a moment; but (as we presume fine weather and a propitious season will be chosen for the event) be carried abroad continually, either in arms or in a carriage, which will divert their minds, and allow them no time to reflect upon their loss, until they become habituated to their new mode of living. It is best, likewise, to keep them awake as much as possible during the day, that they may be inclined to sleep quietly the ensuing night; to aid which important purpose, a gentle anodyne of paregoric, or syrup of white poppies, should be given them at bed-time; as it is very desirable to keep them asleep, if possible, the two or three first nights, after which they will have so far forgot their old habits, as to remain tolerably easy without any artificial means: if not, the anodyne may be repeated without any danger whatever; and is far preferable to letting them cry violently, or contract a habit of getting up, and having a light, which is often productive of lasting inconvenience.

There are various opinions respecting the necessity of permitting infants to drink in the night after we begin to wean them; and many physicians pronounce it not only unnecessary, but impropor. However, I think the health of the child may often be preserved, by suffering them to drink milk once or more for the first few nights, if they are very restless, especially if they have been in the habit of sucking in the night, as is usually the case: otherwise the too sudden change, and going so many hours without food, may have an unkindly effect; but if they sleep quietly, it is certainly best not to begin a practice productive of some trouble.

Some mothers are in the habit of taking the child from the breast in the day-time, and permitting it to suckle in the night preparatory to weaning it; but I think this only prolongs the evil day, for an infant will not be less attached to the breast after a fortnight of such restraint than it was when first refused its favourite food: thus they may be harassed many weeks, when the whole business of weaning might have been over in a few days, and the children equally happy as before.

Many fond mothers revolt at the idea of weaning an infant, lest it should lose that almost exclusive attachment it feels for her while she nurses it, but this will not be the case, provided she is equally attentive to it in every other respect;—the very reverse will generally take place, and the child will appear to cling with redoubled fondness to its remaining friend, as if actuated by the same principle that prompts us in every stage of life, when deprived of a highly valued enjoyment, to cherish with increased anxiety those which are left, and when every earthly comfort is fled, still to look forward to that bright world where the "husband of the widow, and the father of the fatherless,"

"From every eye shall wipe off every tear!"

SECTION II.

Observations on the early Regulation of the infant Temper and Disposition.

> " And should life's olive branches rise
> " To bless your fond parental eyes;
> " SHE who, with all a mother's care,
> " The nursling plants can fondly rear;
> " Th' excrescent shoots with firmness prune,
> " Each noxious weed with care consume,
> " Till, nurtured by her fostering hand,
> " The rising plants grow and expand,
> " Bud, blossom, bear—while each survives
> " The ripened fruits of virtuous lives."
>
> POLYANTHUS.

NAY, do not start my amiable friends, at the intimation that you should begin at eight or nine months old to educate your children; believe me, *now* is the only time to acquire that ascendency over your children's minds, which, if properly employed, will insure you a due degree of influence over them through life. Now, every discreet mother, deeply impressed with the importance of the trust committed to her, will begin by gentle admonition, softened by maternal endearments, to check the first indications of obstinacy and ill temper in her child; for now, like small weeds springing up in a luxuriant soil, they may, *with care*, be easily eradicated; but if permitted by neglect to take root, they will soon overshadow the choicest virtues, or choke them while yet in embryo.

As soon as they can comprehend language, infants may be taught obedience, and their inordinate desires be regulated in such a manner as to prevent their becoming so totally unmanageable, as is too often the case, especially where parents are so unfortunate as to have but one. For instance, should an infant of eight months take a fancy to his mother's diamond watch, as it would be a very improper plaything, he should receive a gentle but *firm* denial; he would probably grieve; something else should then be offered him; if he takes it and is pleased, all will be well; and as often as he reverts to the watch, the denial must be repeated, and he will soon relinquish the expectation, and be perfectly happy with his other toys; and so in every thing else.

On the other hand, should he show resentment when the watch is denied him, and refuse all other playthings that may be offered, instead of weakly yielding to the storm, and with mistaken tenderness giving up the watch, or with anxious care concealing it from his sight, still greater resolution must be observed, tempered with tenderness and moderation, as the object must be to correct the disposition, not to outrage the feelings, and it would be cruel to deny a little creature so alluring an object, and quarrel with him, at *this early age,* for evincing too great a desire for it, before he can be made to reason upon the subject: but on no account permit him to have it, and as often as he inclines to dispute the point, let him perceive you are *determined.* After a few lessons of this kind, your word will no longer be disputed, while your children, thus early taught submission, will never require any severity whatever. But then our government must be uniform to produce this happy effect. It will not do, because we chance to feel out of humour, or it should militate against our own gratifications, to deny an infant an indulgence to-day, which in a paroxysm of maternal fondness, we may grant him to-morrow: believe me, children will very soon learn to take advantage of such capricious conduct; and when once they discover that we are irresolute in our commands, or may be overcome by resolution and importunity on their part, they will not fail to profit by the discovery, and that by such imperceptible degrees, that many a fond mother finds her authority gone, and her jurisdiction contemned, before she is aware that she has by her imbecility forfeited the one, or alienated the other. Nor is this evil confined to infancy. She will feel the melancholy effects of failing to substantiate her claim to obedience from her children during the docile period of childhood, to the latest evening of her life. As the children grow older, the same steady, gentle, but strict discipline, should be observed, avoiding with the most scrupulous care every passionate or abusive epithet. In no one particular do they so soon manifest the image of their great Creator, as in their early sense of justice: therefore, we must be wary, lest, from a desire to crush every vicious propensity in the bud, we accuse them of faults, or censure them for neglect of duty, when they are not guilty, or if guilty, have erred from mistaken, or even praiseworthy motives, as will sometimes happen; for the same sensibility which crimsons the cheek when really in fault, will prompt the ingenuous mind to revolt from unmerited censure, and may leave an impression against us not easily eradicated. If we have reason to suspect a child of a fault of which we have not convincing proof, and cannot by gentle means excite a confession, it is far better to give up the point, and by indirect conversation and remark upon the pernicious effects of such practices, endeavour to impress a due abhorrence of them upon the minds of our little hearers, rather than run the risk of wounding the innocent, by persisting in the accusation. Nor is there the danger some may suppose, of letting the guilty escape by this lenient practice; true, it may sometimes happen, but in general the ingenuous countenance of early childhood will betray the guilty to the penetrating eye of maternal inquiry, provided the inquisitor is actually desirous to discover the truth. But many mothers are so weak as to exclaim within their hearing, when their children are accused, "I know my child never did such a thing in the world—did you my dear?" That child must be a saint indeed, who would not take advantage of so partial a judge, and persist in denying a fact which he perceives his mother determined not to believe. For this reason, as it is of the utmost importance that children should be convinced that their parents will not uphold them in wilful error, they must be led to believe us apprehensive that *they may* be guilty, when charged with a fault, but ready and desirous above every thing to hear them acquit themselves, if possible, and never find us hasty or uncandid in our judgments, nor permit them to suspect us of a determination not to believe them in fault: this is the root of more and greater evils than the contrary extreme. These remarks, however, it must be obvious, relate to an age rather more advanced than that particularly contemplated in this work, although much may and ought to be done during the first two years, that being the time when we must make it our constant care to study and regulate the peculiar tempers and dispositions of our children. These will be manifested and unfolded in a thousand nameless instances, not to be described, which none but a mother can be expected to notice, and which alone can form the criterion by which to regulate the management of them; some infants requiring infinitely more care and pains than others. Thus we frequently see in the same family, one child whom a frown and look of decision will awe into instant obedience; another, whom the least severity will irritate and incense, but who will be gentle as the "shorn lamb," when treated with kindness, and reproved with moderation; one whom the promise of little reward, or the "delicious essence" of well-timed praise, will stimulate to every thing we wish; while nothing short of actual and severe chastisement will have any effect upon another. All these varieties in the infant character, and more also, will be manifest to the critical observer, and should be noted by every one who has the care of children, lest at any time they should wound, by undue severity, the tender and affectionate heart; rouse to anger and resentment the noble and heroic soul; or intimidate and discourage the diffident and humble spirit: or on the other hand, by misplaced indulgence, blind affection, and indiscriminate approbation, confirm a haughty and obstinate temper.

Since so much judgment and discretion is necessary to develope and regulate the infant mind, and form the characters we wish to see adorn the rising generation, " what manner of mothers ought we to be, in all holy conversation and godliness;" or who can wonder at the complaints against ungrateful and disobedient children, or that so many unfortunate parents live to feel

> " How sharper than a serpent's tooth it is
> " To have a thankless child"—

when we reflect how little time the prevailing amusements and habits of fashionable life leave to their fair votaries, for the discharge of their maternal duties, even when their children live beneath the same roof with them, and that many mothers seldom see their infants until brought home from nurse, by which time they have probably acquired many bad habits, and have had none of their natural propensities to evil properly corrected.

 I have one son who very early gave evident signs of an obstinate and passionate temper, of which at nine months old he began to give convincing proof. One day he refused positively for a long time, with every appearance of resentment his age was capable of showing, to take the smallest of two lumps of sugar which had attracted his attention, and which, contrary to my better judgment, I had offered him:—he contended for the large lump: I positively refused; and, perceiving he intended to dispute the point, I thought it a good opportunity to begin to withstand an increasing turbulence of spirit which I had observed with concern from the first dawning of his infant perceptions. Therefore, I determined not to give up, and he went without the sugar until he consented, with a smiling countenance, to take it up from the carpet, where in his anger he had thrown it. I then kissed and praised him, and he seemed conscious he had done something to merit my caresses, and was delighted. Thus began a course of discipline which, in a few years, so entirely subdued a refractory spirit, which bid fair to cause his friends and himself great trouble, that now I have not a more amiable child, or one who renders more prompt obedience to the command of his parents; and this was accomplished before he was four years old, so that I have had no occasion to use the least severity since. I mention this as an instance to enforce my favourite maxim, that it is far better, by gentle and steady government, to subdue an untoward temper in infancy, than be compelled to greater severity in a few years, or permit our children to grow up the slaves of their passions and desires, to curse in after life that indiscriminate indulgence, which must end in constant disappointment and vexation, if not utter ruin. Indeed, I very much doubt, if parents do not properly subdue the tempers of their children within the first two or three years, whether it is ever done afterwards, except by bitter adversity, which will often have a contrary effect, and drive the unhappy child of injudicious, unprincipled fondness *to despair*, when, if he had been early taught the great duties of self-denial and submission to the divine will, he would have buffeted the storm with the strong sinews of resolution and conscious duty, and, sheltered by the broad mantle of resignation to the dispensations of an allwise Providence, rose superior to every affliction.

The great error in infant management arises from an idea many well meaning parents entertain, that the little creatures must be indulged in all their whims and wishes, however inconvenient to their friends, or injurious to themselves, until they grow old enough to reason about right and wrong: on the contrary, children should never know the time when they are permitted to have their uncontrolled will in any thing, but should always be taught to consider every indulgence, however trivial, a favour. A mother's government should begin so early, and continue so uniformly, that they shall never know the time when she did not have undisputed sway. When this is not the case, they acquire almost imperceptibly a thousand factitious wants and ungovernable desires, which at length grow so intolerable, that even the parents lose their patience, and then the children must be beaten, or constantly thwarted in their caprices, now become innumerable, and thus prove the little torments of the whole family, destroying all peace and comfort wherever they appear, and finally rendering parents and guests perfectly unhappy. How melancholy this picture, and how great the pity that we see it so often exhibited. Let it then be amongst the earliest impressions received by the infant mind, that you know what is best for them, and are determined to consult their good, without attending to their whims, or weakly yielding to their impetuous tempers, and you will quickly reverse the picture entirely, and harmony, peace and happiness shine resplendent round your dwellings. Yet I am far from agreeing with many learned writers on the subject of infant education, who assert that we should never permit our children to persuade us to alter our decisions, or, when once we have passed our word either for or against them, suffer any consideration to induce us to retract. This appears so contrary to every principle of justice, that I think it cannot be right. A child, for instance, may ask a favour, which on the first view appears very improper: consequently, we refuse to grant it; but upon inquiry, or more mature reflection, we become convinced that it is not only proper, but for the child's best interest that it should be indulged. Shall we in this case adhere to our first decision, and grieve the heart of a little dependent being, whom we have taught to know that from us there is no appeal, merely because we have pronounced our fiat, without any regard whatever to the feelings of the aggrieved party. I am convinced children very early discover such a just sense of right and wrong, as will revolt at such arbitrary government, and that they will feel greater respect, and *infinitely* more affection, for a mother who will candidly confess she was too hasty, and exert herself to repair the injury they may have sustained. Nor will her ready acquiescence in this case lessen her authority in the least, provided the child perceives it proceeds from a conviction of the propriety of the request, and not merely from a blind indulgence to its wishes, or an inability to resist importunity.

Those writers, however, argue that we must be ever on our guard, and never give an unjust denial or hasty reproof. If I mistake not, the elegant author of Cœlebs in search of a Wife, makes the excellent Mr. Stanley advance some such a sentiment. Had every mother the perfections which are so captivatingly displayed in that inimitable character, happy indeed would it be for the rising generation; but I fear they rarely fall to the lot of mothers, surrounded by a numerous offspring, whose clashing interests and wants call for continual interference, where even her maternal tenderness will often throw her off her guard, and prompt a hasty decision, "more honoured in the breach than the observance:" nevertheless, we shall all do well to keep so bright a star in view, and follow it as nearly as possible until we arrive at our journey's end, and receive the rich reward of all our toils.

I have thus far touched upon this important subject, although somewhat foreign to the purpose of this little volume, as I esteem the health of the mind of even greater importance than the health of the body: and indeed they are, as it respects infants, very intimately connected; for what mother can vouch for the health of her babe a single hour, if she has not command enough over herself and him to control his appetites, wants and desires; on the due regulation of which, not only his happiness but his health must depend.

I was here almost tempted to address a word or two of advice to *fathers;* but my own good man, who sits laughing on the sofa, whilst his favourite little Joseph is drawing his watch tied to a string round the carpet for a plaything, and who just now *looked* as if he thought me cruel for refusing the dear enchanting little innocent my inkstandish for a go-cart, might esteem it too *presuming*.

CHAPTER IV.

SECTION I.

On the Diseases to which Children are peculiarly subject at this Age.

> " Sickness, the minister of death, doth lay
> " So strong a siege against our brittle clay,
> " As while it doth our weak forts singly win,
> " It hopes at length to take all mankind in :
> " First it begins upon the womb to wait,
> " And doth the unborn child there uncreate,
> " Then rocks the cradle where the infant lies,
> " Where, ere it fully be alive, it dies."
>
> CAREW.

It is now proper, according to my original design, to give some few directions for the treatment of those common complaints, to which every child is subject during the first years of its existence, and few fail sooner or later to experience. For those complicated disorders which require the judgment and the skill of a Harvey or a Cullen, it would be equally presumptuous in me to prescribe, or my fair readers to practise my prescriptions. I shall therefore confine myself to very narrow limits, and speak only of such complaints as I frequently manage successfully in my own family, and which every lady ought to understand enough to administer the first remedies, by which she may often save herself many groundless alarms, and her children much suffering.

Some physicians assert that women never ought to open a medical book, or presume to meddle with medical knowledge in the least, lest they become fanciful, and conceit themselves and families ill with every disease they read of: not so the celebrated Dr. Buchan; and while we venerate him for his philanthropy, and zeal for the diffusion of professional knowledge, we must admire and honour his candour and humanity. He thus speaks upon this important subject:

"People are told, that if they dip the least into medical knowledge, it will render them fanciful, and make them believe they have got every disease of which they read. Perhaps this may be the case with those who are fanciful beforehand. But suppose it were so with others, they must be soon undeceived. A short time will show them their error, and a little more reading will infallibly correct it. A single instance will show the absurdity of this notion. A sensible lady, rather than read a medical performance, which would instruct her in the management of her children, must leave them entirely to the care and conduct of the most ignorant, credulous, and superstitious part of the human species." And again, when endeavouring to impress upon the minds of our sex the great importance of the truly maternal character, he has this impressive passage: "Did mothers reflect on their own importance, and lay it to heart, they would embrace every opportunity of informing themselves of the duties they owe their infant offspring. It is their province not only to form the body, but also to give the mind its most early bias. They have it very much in their power to make men healthy or valetudinary, useful in life, or the pests of society." Such sentiments from the pen of a physician of eminence, must have great weight with every mother who is anxious to discharge the sacred duties of her station. Every lady will be sensible of the truth of the position in the passage first quoted, if she will but read, and study, and learn, "How fearfully and wonderfully we are made," and thereby qualify herself to mitigate the sufferings of her fellow creatures in a manner not practicable by the multitude: any one may bestow money—it is " trash"—

"'Tis his, 'twas mine, and has been slave to thousands;"

but it is the privilege of the benevolent matron to extend the cooling draught to the parched lips of poverty and sickness, and smooth the cradle of the panting infant, while directing the grateful mother how to restore the little sufferer to health; and thus diffuse the balm of hope through the dwellings of indigence and sorrow.

It is my sincere wish that this little volume may prove a useful assistant to this beneficent work, by furnishing my readers with a concise and simple statement of the charac-

P

teristic symptoms of the various complaints to which children are subject, in so small a compass, that it may become a pocket companion, always at hand, and always faithful. Therefore, I shall endeavour to render it so far scientific, by quotations from respectable medical authors, as will enable every intelligent reader to proceed with confidence when called upon to administer the cordial or the drug, for the relief of any complaint here specified, and with the aid of the rules given in note (1), they may portion out the medicines required with exactness; which is of the utmost importance.

The better to promote the end desired, every lady who has a family, or who wishes to impart the blessings of her medical knowledge to her poor neighbours, should furnish herself with a medicine chest, containing every drug of known and established efficacy, and a set of scales and weights proper for the purpose; for no one but a regularly bred physician should ever venture to give any potent drug, especially opium, calomel, or emetic tartar, unless weighed with scrupulous exactness, according to the above-mentioned rules. If thus provided, she may become a blessing to the community around her, at an expense comparatively trivial. One of the most distressing disorders of which I shall speak, is

The Dysentery.

Under the heads of teething, and the diseases of the first months, I said all that is requisite in a work of this nature, on the common relaxes to which infants are liable; but the dysentery being much more distressing in its effects upon the human body, I think it calls for the first place in a book purposely intended to assist the anxious mother, when her children are taken suddenly ill, and no better assistance can be procured. The dysentery usually comes on with all the symptoms of a fever, such as pain in the head and back, shivering, nausea, and sometimes vomiting, extreme pain in the bowels, and total loss of appetite, attended with great weakness and universal debility; so that children who can speak, will usually complain that they are tired and cannot stand; and an infant in arms, when not in extreme pain, will appear weak and languid, and lie almost stupid, or be very restless and seem in universal distress. Sometimes patients will have a very flushed face and high fever, and others will be pale and cadaverous, their eyes sunk, and their whole countenance changed. But the most *characteristic* symptoms of this dreadful disease, is the distressing *tenesmus* which constantly attends it, and destroys all possibility of rest, until we can succeed in removing it. When, from all or any of these symptoms, there is reason to think the dysentery has occurred, the first step is to clear out the first passages; for this purpose an emetic of ipecacuanha must be given: after it begins to operate, the patient should drink freely of chamomile tea, the antiseptic qualities of which are peculiarly adapted to the nature of this disease; a gentle opiate should be given at bed-time, and repeated in the course of the night every three hours, if the tenesmus and other distressing symptoms do not abate, and the patient rest quietly without. The next day a dose of rhubarb and calomel, or calomel alone, must be administered. If simple calomel is preferred, castor oil should be given in about three hours, the quantities to be regulated according to the age of the child, by the rule before mentioned. If this medicine has the desired effect, as it often will, the little patients will regain their appetites in some measure, and ask for food: great care must then be taken to prevent their eating any thing improper; animal food, and fish of all kinds, and every thing inclined to putrefaction, should be strictly avoided, as the bowels are already too much disposed to mortification : therefore, every thing we give either as food or medicine, should tend to carry off the offensive contents of the stomach and bowels, and sheath, strengthen, and heal the intestines. Mutton, or chicken broth, with rice boiled in it, calves-foot jellies, plain light puddings, custards, milk, with rice or the grated flour boiled in it, are all good, and may be offered in succession; for it is very desirable in this disorder to procure something that the patient can relish, and that will set upon the stomach: when that is accomplished, and the appetite returns, a cure is almost certain, without the aid of any more medicine. The drink should be tea made of any of the mucilaginous herbs, such as marsh mallows, *cudwort,* which is most excellent, and is said to effect a cure sometimes of itself. The roots and leaves of the running blackberry is particularly recommended; flax seed and hyssop is also very good, where there is much fever; and these may all be tried alternately, if the disease proves obstinate. At the commencement of the disorder, the patient's feet should be bathed in warm water, and drafts applied to them, and renewed as often as they grow dry. Where burdock leaves are to be had, they should be preferred to every thing else for this purpose: let the fresh leaves be gathered, and the large stalks cut off, then lay them upon a table and roll them with a kitchen rolling pin, then hold them to the fire until they wilt and become soft and pliable: in this state bind them round the feet: they are excellent in all putrid febrile disorders: where they cannot be procured, the garlic drafts already mentioned may be used; or if those are not to be had, mustard seed boiled in vinegar and made into a paste with rye flour will answer, care being taken that they are not made too strong, or they will blister the tender feet of an infant. The bathing and drafts should be renewed twice a day until the disorder is conquered. The elixir paregoric (2) should be given as often as once in two or three hours while the pain and tenesmus continue, to procure the unfortunate little patient as much rest as possible, and allay the spasms and irritation to which infants and young children are so peculiarly liable.

The bed, chamber, and every thing about the sick person, should be kept extremely clean, and its linen changed every day, as in all disorders tending to putrescence, it is very detrimental to permit the little frame, already loaded with disease, to imbibe again the bad humours kind nature is struggling to expel from the innumerable pores of the skin; which will infallibly happen, unless the clothes worn next the body are frequently changed. The greatest care should be taken to have them all perfectly dry and well aired, as damp clothes, beds, &c. are said to be among the usual causes of the dysentery. A current of fresh air should be allowed to pass constantly through the room, (if the patient is so ill as to be confined,) but if possible they should be carried abroad every day; and if they reside in the city, or a populous town, they should be removed as soon as possible to the country, where they may enjoy abundant exercise in a fresh and pure air. The first care of parents, who have a large family of children in a neighbourhood where the dysentery prevails, should be to remove them as soon as possible beyond the reach of infection, as few diseases are more contagious: if this is impracticable, the next object is to prevent the ill consequences, by fumigating the room frequently with burning vinegar, or other sharp acid, and scenting the bed, pillows, and every thing about the room, with essences of tansy, spear-mint, rue, lavender, or any other strong aromatic herb.

By practices similar to the above, I have succeeded in restoring several of my little ones to health, when afflicted with this cruel disorder, and never had it prevail through my family. However, for the satisfaction of those ladies who may live at a great distance from approved medical aid, I will extract some passages from **Dr.** Wallis and **Dr.** Buchan upon the treatment of it. **Dr.** Wallis, after describing at large the various kinds of dysentery, which he divides into three distinct kinds, the "*inflammatory kind,*" where there will be a high degree of fever; the "*putrid kind,*" where the feverish symptoms are slight, the face pale, &c.; and the "*malignant sort,*" where there is little fever, but the patient in more danger than in either of the other cases, goes on to say: "Of whatever nature this disease may be, the indications are similar, and depend upon evacuating the acrimony, or determining it to other places, weakening its action, alleviating the distressing symptoms, by rendering the intestines less sensible to its irritating effects in *its first stages;* in the *last,* recovering the tone, and giving strength to the relaxed and weakened vessels. To promote these purposes, in full habits, where there are apparent symptoms of inflammation, the patient should be bled once or twice, according to their urgency, and the strength of the patient. In the next place, the stomach and intestines should be unloaded by emetics and cathartics; twelve grains of powdered ipecacuanha, and one of tartarized antimony, should be well mixed together, and divided into three parts, and one given every second hour; no liquid should be taken after the first dose; but after the third, weak beef tea, or chicken broth, should be drank liberally, to encourage the vomiting, after which a slight opiate will be requisite. Should the emetic produce smart evacuations upwards and downwards the succeeding day, it is not necessary to order any thing except a grain of opium, mixed with three or four grains of ipecacuanha into pills, with syrup of white poppy heads, and given at bed-time. But, should the emetic not have produced any purgative effects, a purging powder, made of thirty grains of rhubarb and three of calomel, must be administered the morning following. As for my own part, in the beginning of this complaint I prefer the castor oil emulsion (3), as it relaxes the coats of the stomach, sheathes the acrimony, produces evacuations, and mitigates the pains of the bowels. But as is the nature of the disease, so should be the election of our purgatives. If of the inflammatory kind, the *salines* are preferable; if the putrescent, the antiseptic, as tamarinds, cream of tartar, &c.; but in every case, after the effect is produced, an opiate should be administered at night. In the intermediate spaces of time, small doses of nitre, accompanied with antimonials and saline mixtures, may be exhibited, joined with sheathing medicines, such as gum tragacanth, arabic, starch, if the fever keeps up; or should it be of the *low malignant*, gentle cordials are proper. However, should not the disease soon yield to this mode, but the symptoms still continue, particularly griping and purging, small doses of ipecacuanha may be given, sufficient only to create a nausea, increasing or decreasing the dose agreeably to the effects, and joining it with antiseptics (4), cooling, or cordial medicines, as the case may require. Should the stools continue remarkably viscid and offensive, every second or third day a purgative should be given, and at night an opiate. We must proceed in this manner, till, from the regularity of the pulse, the cessation of pain, and propensity to stools, as well as from the want of them, we may conclude the disease terminated; but should not these appearances occur in the course of a few days, we have reason to apprehend the greatest danger: we must then, if the symptoms continue as violent as at first, have recourse to fomentations, and clysters of the sheathing and anodyne sort, made of milk, broth, marsh mallow, or linseed decoction, with starch and tincture of opium.

"Besides the ipecacuanha, other medicines are recommended, and, if we believe the recommendation, falling little short of infallibility; namely, from two to ten grains of created glass of antimony; from ten to fifteen grains of powdered columbo, every three or four hours: the decoction of semirauba bark is considered as a specific, and said to remove the disease without the danger or inconveniences attendant on astringents.

"At the close of the complaint, astringents are useful, particularly tonics; and indeed, also when the most violent symptoms of fever, pain, and tenesmus have ceased, to relieve the relaxed state of the vessels. In pursuing the modes here laid down, we shall seldom fail of curing this complaint; but should it be accompanied with a putrid malignant fever, there will be little hope of recovery. However, we should try the effects of antiseptics, particularly wine, infusions of bark and snake root, with a few drops of tincture of opium in each dose, and the free use of sub-acid fruits, taken by themselves, or squeezed plentifully into other liquors. Indeed, fruit, and things of a similar nature, will form, in these cases, the proper plan of diet; but when dysenteries are unattended with any high degree of putrefaction, decoctions, and jellies of rice, sago, tapioca, salep, the white decoction, chalk mixture, weak chicken broth or beef tea, are most proper; though all solid animal food must be avoided.

" When flatulencies become distressing, which will sometimes be the case, chamomile flower tea, infusion of cinnamon or cloves, or liquids, impregnated slightly with other aromatics, may be occasionally administered with great advantage.

" With respect to the *common diarrhœa,* if it is unattended with any weakness, loss of appetite, or febrile affections, and is moderate in quantity, it very often is of service to the constitution, and is rather conducive to health than otherwise; but should it run on to too great excess, it will require the same means for its cure, and will be conquered much more easily than the dysentery; and, indeed, all the other species we have specified require the same treatment; at the beginning, clearing the first passages of any irritating contents by proper emetics and cathartics; next, soliciting the flow of fluids to the surface by diaphoretics, and strengthening the stomach and bowels by tonic astringents, bitters, strengthening medicines, and *particularly* riding on horseback, at the close of the disease."

These directions are so full and satisfactory that, methinks, almost any person might undertake the cure of the complaint with so good a guide, where the medicines could be procured. It must be remembered, however, by my fair readers, that the doses, &c. are calculated for adults, and, therefore, must be proportioned by the standard given us by Dr. Underwood.

Dr. Buchan differs so little in the mode of cure that it is unnecessary to recapitulate the particulars; he has, however, some remarks upon regimen which may be of use. His directions as to cleanliness, air, exercise, and diet, are almost the same as may be found in the first part of this article. " A flannel waistcoat worn next the skin, has often a very good effect in the dysentery. This promotes the perspiration without overheating the body. Great caution, however, is necessary in leaving it off. I have known a dysentery brought on by imprudently throwing off a flannel waistcoat before the season was sufficiently warm. For whatever purpose this piece of dress is worn, it should never be left off but in a warm season. In a putrid dysentery, the patient may be allowed to eat freely of most kinds of good ripe fruit; as apples, grapes, currants, strawberries, &c.; these may either be eat raw or boiled with or without milk, as the patient chooses. The prejudices against fruit in this disease are so great, that many believe it to be the common cause of dysenteries; this, however, is an egregious mistake; both reason and experience show that good fruit is one of the best medicines both for the prevention and cure of the dysentery.

" The most proper drink is whey. The dysentery has often been cured by the use of clear whey alone. It may be taken both for drink and in form of clyster. When whey cannot be had, barley-water, sharpened with cream of tartar, may be drank; or, a decoction of barley and tamarinds; two ounces of the former and one of the latter, may be boiled in two English quarts of water to one.

"Chamomile tea, if the stomach will bear it, is an exceeding proper drink; it both strengthens the stomach, and, by its antiseptic quality, tends to prevent a mortification of the bowels."

The chief variation as to medicine, in the directions given by these two physicians, is the substitution of calomel and oily emulsions in Dr. Wallis's practice, for rhubarb only, which is recommended by Dr. Buchan; and from what little experience I have had, I must acknowledge myself in favour of calomel and castor oil, in this complaint, for young children especially: it is less nauseous, and the stomach is so very irritable few children can keep the rhubarb down; and, although it is a principle with me to begin very early to habituate them to take their medicine without hesitation, yet common humanity will dictate the desire to choose the least disagreeable of two drugs, when they are equally efficacious; and, indeed, I believe, calomel is esteemed the best in all diarrhœtic complaints by many modern practitioners of high respectability. I have found molasses and water a most excellent drink in this disorder, and it is said to be best to pour boiling water upon the molasses and let it cool; but I fancy this is immaterial. When the appetite returns, the gingerbread before-mentioned is as good an article of food as can well be prepared to forward the curative intention. I once had a child very ill with the dysentery, who eat very little else for several days, and recovered surprisingly fast.

When we have succeeded in procuring ease to our little patient, and the distressing tenesmus and excruciating pain are gone, we must not think all danger over, and our attentions no longer necessary. The utmost care is still requisite to perfect a cure, as children once affected with this disorder are very subject to a relapse, which too often proves fatal. Therefore, the most scrupulous attention to the diet must be observed, letting it still consist altogether of milk, fruits, broth, and jellies, with plain light bread and puddings: and, also, that they have constant exercise in the open air, either in a carriage or on horseback. This, and the tender attentions of a fond mother, can scarcely fail to restore the little *invalid to health*.

Worms.

These vexatious vermin are often the source of innumerable complaints in children, from the time they are weaned, and sometimes before, until the age of puberty. Those infants who have been indulged in promiscuous feeding from the birth, are most apt to be afflicted by them, which should be an additional inducement to mothers not to permit the pernicious practice. I recollect visiting a poor woman in my neighbourhood, some years ago, who sent for me to comfort her beneath one of the greatest afflictions the human heart can sustain, a lovely and beloved child lay expiring in the cradle, totally insensible to all around, in which distressing condition it had continued for several days, and now all hope was over. The physicians judged its disorder to proceed from worms, and a vast number had been evacuated, but without producing any good effect. I asked the disconsolate mother, if the child had always been subject to them; she replied in the affirmative, but added, "She has always been a very hearty child, and wanted to eat every thing ever since she was two months old." I asked her if she did not think it hurtful for infants to eat *every thing;* she replied, "she did not know but it was, but she could never deny the dear little creature any thing she had; and now, (added she, while her eyes streamed with tears,) now I have the comfort of reflecting, she always had every thing she wanted!" What mistaken fondness! I recollected to have seen the child when in health, and noticed its uncommon florid countenance; I was no longer at a loss to account for this, or its sudden and fatal illness. Butter, and all fat and oily aliments, are said to be very injurious to children who are predisposed to worms. But as my family have been remarkably free from them, I shall not pretend to direct from my own experience.

but furnish my readers with advice from the rich stores of learning and skill, from which I have already made large drafts. Dr. Buchan thus describes the different kinds, causes, and modes of cure:

"These are chiefly of three kinds, viz. the *tænia* or tape-worm; the *teres*, or round and long worm; and the *ascarides*, or round and short worm. The long round worms occasion squeamishness, vomiting, and disagreeable breath, gripes, looseness, swelling of the belly, swooning, loathing of food, and, at other times, a voracious appetite, a dry cough, convulsions, epileptic fits, and sometimes a privation of speech. These worms have been known to perforate the intestines, and get into the cavity of the belly. The effects of the tape worm are the same as the long and round, but rather more violent.

"The round worms, called ascarides, besides an itching, cause swooning and tenesmus.

"Andry says, the following symptoms particularly attend the *solium*, which is a species of the tape worm, viz. swoonings, privation of speech, and a voracious appetite.

"*Causes.* Worms may proceed from various causes; but they are seldom found except in weak and relaxed stomachs, where the digestion is bad. Sedentary persons are more liable to them, than the active and laborious. Those who eat great quantities of unripe fruit, or who live much on raw herbs and roots, are generally subject to worms. They are often a symptom of fevers and other acute diseases. There seems to be a hereditary disposition in some persons to this disease. I have often seen all the children of a family subject to worms of a particular kind. They seem likewise frequently owing to the nurse. Children of the same family, nursed by one woman, have often worms, when those nursed by another have none. Children are more liable to this disease than adults; though infants on the breast are seldom troubled with it. To this, however, there are several exceptions. I have seen a child who passed worms before it was three months old. They were, indeed, of a very particular kind, being real caterpillars: some of them were above an inch long; they had red heads, and were so brisk as to jump about; they lived several days after the child had passed them. Another child, suckled by the same woman, passed the same kind of worms while upon the breast. Both children suffered extremely before the worms came away.

"*Symptoms.* The common symptoms of worms are, paleness of countenance, and, at other times, a universal flushing of the face; itching of the nose: this, however, is doubtful, as children pick their noses in all diseases; starting and grinding of the teeth in sleep; swelling of the upper lip; the appetite sometimes bad, and at other times very voracious; looseness; a sour, or stinking breath; a hard swelled belly; great thirst; the urine frothy, and sometimes of a whitish colour; an involuntary discharge of *saliva*, especially when asleep; frequent pains of the side, with a dry cough and unequal pulse; palpitations of the heart; swoonings; drowsiness; cold sweats; palsy; epileptic fits; with many other unaccountable nervous symptoms, which were formerly attributed to witchcraft, or the influence of evil spirits. Small bodies in the excrements resembling melon or cucumber seeds are symptoms of the tape worm. I lately saw some very surprising effects of worms in a girl about five years of age, who used to lie whole hours as if dead. She at last expired, and upon opening her body a number of the *teres*, or long round worms, were found in her guts, which were very much inflamed; and what anatomists call an *intersusceptio*, or involving of one part of the gut within another, had taken place in no less than four different parts of the intestinal canal.

"*Medicines.* For a child of four or five years old, ten grains of rhubarb, five of jalap, and two of calomel, may be mixed in a spoonful of syrup or honey, and given in the morning. The child should keep the house all day, and take nothing cold. This dose may be repeated *twice a week* for *three* or *four* weeks. On the intermediate days the child may take a scruple of powdered tin, and ten grains of æthiops mineral in a spoonful of treacle twice a-day. These doses must be increased or diminished according to the age of the patient. Bisset says, the great bastard black hellebore or bearsfoot, is a most powerful vermifuge for the long round worm. He orders the decoction of about a drachm of the green leaves, or about fifteen grains of the dried leaves, in powder, for a dose for a child betwixt four and seven years of age. This dose is to be repeated two or three times. He adds, that the green leaves made into a syrup, with coarse sugar, is almost the only medicine he has used for round worms for three years past. Before pressing out the juice he moistens the leaves with vinegar, which corrects the medicine. The dose is a tea-spoonful at bed-time, and one or two next morning.

" I have frequently known those big bellies, which in children are commonly reckoned a sign of worms, quite removed by giving them white soap in their pottage or other food. Tansy, garlic, and rue, are all good against worms, and may be used in various ways. We might here mention many other plants both for internal and external use; but think the powder of tin with æthiops mineral, and the purges of rhubarb and calomel, are more to be depended on. Ball's purging vermifuge powder is a very powerful medicine; it is made of equal parts of rhubarb, scammony, and calomel, with as much double refined sugar as is equal to the weight of all the other ingredients. These must be well mixed together, and reduced to a fine powder. The dose for a child is from ten grains to twenty, once or twice a week. Parents who would preserve their children from worms must allow them plenty of exercise in the open air; to take care that their food be wholesome and sufficiently solid; and, as far as possible, to prevent their eating raw herbs, roots, or green trashy fruits. It will not be amiss to allow a child who is subject to worms a glass of red wine after meals; as every thing that braces and strengthens the stomach is good both for preventing and expelling these vermin." In a note we find the following salutary caution.

"We think it necessary here to warn people of their danger, who buy cakes, powders, and other worm medicines, at random, from quacks, and give them to their children without proper care. The principal ingredients in most of these medicines is mercury, which is never to be trifled with. I lately saw a shocking instance of the danger of this conduct. A girl who had taken a dose of worm powder, bought of a travelling quack, went out, and, perhaps, was so imprudent as to drink cold water, during its operation. She immediately swelled, and died that very day, with all the symptoms of having been poisoned."

Dr. Wallis mentions tansy as an anthelmintic, tending to strengthen the stomach and bowels, and give tone and activity to the intestines; he also mentions *sabine,* worm-seed, Indian pink root in powder, fern root powder, and many other simples, as being of service in worm complaints, but concludes with observing, "that calomel is one of our most superior vermifuges," to which I sincerely assent, as far as my experience has enabled me to judge: however, when children are afflicted with the long round worms, they will sometimes rise in the stomach and throat, and cause very alarming symptoms, and not unfrequently convulsion fits; it is then found very beneficial to macerate the leaves of double tansy; either dry or fresh will answer, in a little spirits

over a gentle heat until soft, then put the
leaves so moistened into a little bag, and apply
it just *above* the pit of the stomach; this will
usually prevent the recurrence of the distressing symptoms, and give the child great relief;
the essence of tansy dropped on sugar, children in general are fond of, and it should be
given every morning, and again before dinner,
to those who are subject to worms, whenever
they begin to show indications of any indisposition which can reasonably be attributed to
them; the essence of peppermint is equally
good, and may be used in the same way; indeed, it is often preferable when loss of appetite is a symptom. I have a little girl who
appeared very unwell last spring, would look
extremely pale in the morning, and had no
appetite for her breakfast; from a very bad
breath, and some other circumstances, I con-
cluded worms were the exciting cause of her
ill health. I immediately began (after being
convinced that air, exercise, and regimen,
failed of the desired effect,) to give her the
essence above recommended, and in half an
hour after taking her dose in the morning she

would have a fine appetite, and eat her bread and milk with the keenest relish, and in six weeks time all her faint languid symptoms disappeared, and now she enjoys fine health, and can scarcely wait until the servant brings her breakfast after she rises. It should always be remembered, by every one who has the care of children, that medicine does not work by magic, and therefore cannot be expected to cure any complaint instantaneously. It is the mistaken idea that a medicine which does not cure immediately will never cure, that so often renders the best advice and most appropriate treatment abortive: it frequently happens also that we give some drug which very soon procures a mitigation of the symptoms; we then think nature will do the rest, and remit the medicine; the disease returns with renewed energy, like a baffled enemy, who, perceiving his opponent off his guard, or wholly withdrawn, returns to the attack with renovated courage, confident of victory: and so it too frequently happens; the second attack is worse than the first. We should, therefore, when we find a medicine beneficial to any complaint whatever, persevere in the use of it until the cure is performed, or, we are convinced by candid and sufficient experiment, that it is not equal alone to the conquest of the disease. It is a well known fact, especially in eruptive complaints, that a remedy which is actually adequate to the cure, will make the disorder apparently worse at first, by throwing it out of the blood upon the surface, which is evidently the true indication, but which many persons who do not reflect upon the nature of the case, look upon as a bad symptom, and abandon the medicine from a supposition that it makes them worse. This is an error, which, it is hoped, more general information as to the nature and effects of medicine on the frame would happily correct. The happy effect of the simple medicine above-mentioned on my little girl, was not produced in a day nor a week; I gave it to her every morning, or every other morning, for several weeks.

I have heard some ladies express a fear of giving an emetic in worm complaints, lest it should cause them to rise in the stomach and occasion fits or suffocation; but I have been assured, by very able physicians, that this is a mistaken idea, for if the worms were actually in the stomach they ought to be brought away, and then an emetic might be of service, or, indeed, the only remedy; but if they were not in the stomach, taking an emetic would never bring them into that bowel, especially ipecacuanha, for they loath all bitter or nauseous drugs. Therefore, whenever my children are seized with vomiting or nausea, or have high feverish symptoms, which I have reason to attribute to worms, and they will not yield to light, cordial, or aromatic medicines, I immediately give them an emetic of ipecac or antimonial wine, and the following day some purgative medicine: by this means fevers are often prevented, and if worms are the exciting cause, they will probably be evacuated in the course of the operation; and if the child is not materially better after it is over, the indication is obvious; some more powerful vermifuge must be resorted to immediately.

Measles.

This disease is thus described by Dr. Wallis: " According to my conception, it is in general a febrile disease of the inflammatory kind, always infectious, electively affecting that membrane called scheiderian, which lines the inside of the nose, throat and lungs, and, in its progression, the skin; though I have seen the affection of the lungs so extremely slight, as not to call forth the least attention, where there was a diarrhœa attended through the whole course of the disease. Its progress is divided into three stages; the *first* precedes, the *second* attends, and the *last* succeeds the completion of the eruption. At the commencement, there are chillness and heat alternately succeeding each other; soon after, on the second day, the fever increases, attended with considerable sickness, great heat, thirst, languor, and loss of appetite; the tongue is white; there is a heaviness of the head and drowsiness, sneezing, brightness of the eyes, from whence flow a thin humour; the eyelids swell, and most commonly there is a dry and very troublesome cough; sometimes vomiting and looseness are associates with these; the last of a dark green colour, when children are getting their teeth; and all these symptoms gradually increase, till the *eruptive* or *secondary* stage begins, which occurs generally on the fourth day, about which time small red spots, like flea bites, make their appearance on the face, which run into clusters, forming larger spots, rising above the skin, perceptible only to the touch, not to the sight; afterwards broad spots spread over the body downwards, not quite so prominent, though of a higher colour than those of the face: when the eruption is finished the vomiting ceases, but the fever increases; and the cough, with the difficulty of breathing, becomes more violent; a sweat and diarrhœa now and then supervene.

" On the sixth day, or thereabout, the *third stage* begins, on which the spots on the face grow dry, and give it a rough appearance; and in three days more they totally disappear from the whole body; for on the ninth day nothing is to be seen, except a dark coloured fine farina, or appearance like bran, all over the surface of the skin: at this period, the fever and cough are sometimes alleviated, sometimes increased, and terminate in a dangerous peripneumony, and not unfrequently a looseness succeeds the disease.

" After this we are not to conclude the patient out of danger, unless, during its course, some considerable evacuation has taken place, either by sweating, vomiting, urine, or looseness; for without something of this kind occurs, the cough will continue, the fever will return with additional violence, and the strength not be recovered except with great commotion in the system, and, consequently, extreme danger.

"Though what we have here described is the most frequent mode of the measles appearance and progress, to their termination, yet sometimes they differ so much that authors have denominated them *anomalous,* or *irregular,* as deviating from the common course, or as in the eruption putting on the appearance of the small-pox.

Characteristic signs. An infectious inflammatory fever for the most part, with which are associated a defluxion of a thin watery humour from the eyes, tickling in the nose, sneezing, dry cough, more or less violent; on the fourth day, sometimes sooner, sometimes later, though rarely, small spots running together, perceptible to the touch on the face, but broader on the body, not perceptibly elevated above the skin, break forth, which in three days after are converted into branny scales in part, and totally disappear upon the ninth day.

" *Cure.* In so mild a manner will the measles sometimes affect patients, that little is necessary to be done, except abstinence from all *animal food*, or heating applications; and drinking freely of thin watery acessent liquids, such as common fig drink, made agreeably acid with lemon-juice, apple water, or some such like fluids. But should the febrile symptoms run high, we must proceed as directed in the small-pox; but great attention must be paid to the affection of the lungs; oily emulsions and tinctures, may therefore be prescribed occasionally in conjunction with the other remedies, calculated to keep the febrile affections within proper limits.

"Should oily medicines disagree with the stomach, as is sometimes the case, we must have recourse to the class of demulcents, using the pectoral decoction, or that of linseed, as common drink.

"After the eruption is completed, slight opiates are serviceable; but as nature generally performs her crisis either by sweats, looseness, or urine, we must observe what way she directs her efforts, and proceed as we have before directed in cures of this kind, where they occur in fevers not eruptive.

"As soon as the redness of the skin goes off, and the spots begin to die away, gentle purgatives must be administered, at proper intervals, and the patient return to his usual mode of life gradually. Care also should be taken that patients expose not themselves too early to the cold air; for these are apt to bring on a very disagreeable cough, asthma, and consumption, from affections of the lungs, or of some other parts."

Much more is said by this learned author

upon the variations in the measles, enumerating many distressing aspects sometimes assumed by this disease; but as I am not writing with an idea to make physicians, but merely to enable my readers to *nurse* their infants with the aid of the physician, or *prescribe* for them in slight and ordinary attacks, I shall not transcribe more on this subject, except one paragraph, which, I think, merits attention from the faculty in general.

" Few people have thought the measles to be a disease of sufficient consequence, to avail themselves of those assistances, which, as in the small-pox, might be derived from inoculation in this complaint. As for my own part, *practically*, I cannot say any thing on the subject; but if we may believe the authority of some who have made the experiment, or be allowed to depend on reasoning from analogy, our labours might be happily rewarded; for it is asserted, and appears probable, that from inoculation from infected blood, on the sixth day a slight fever manifests itself most commonly, though it is very moderate, unattended with loss of sleep and inflammatory symptoms; and it is neither succeeded by a hectic fever, cough, nor inflamed eyes; so that we find we should be freed from a train of the most dangerous symptoms, and consequently relieved, in many cases, from the most distressing apprehensions."

Surely the experiment is worth trying, provided it is unattended with danger, which appears to be the case. All my children except the three youngest had this disease at the same time, and very favourably; they were not confined but a day or two, each one; indeed, some of them were able to go about the house during the whole course of the disease, although very feeble. The physician who attended them, treated the disease upon the same plan as he would have done the smallpox, in opposition to the ancient method of keeping the patients in bed from fear of their taking cold, and thereby increasing the defluxion, cough, &c. After two or three days, while the eruption was coming out, my children were able to run about, and disposed to play, in which they were indulged, and they recovered surprisingly fast; the cough left them with the other symptoms, and no ill consequences whatever occurred. Children in general, I believe, have the disease lighter than adults, partly from their youth, but chiefly from their simple manner of living, and regular habits.

It is a practice with me, whenever any of my family are seized with feverish symptoms for which I cannot readily account, to give them a draught of *saffron tea,* to defend the stomach in case the disease should prove eruptive; and I am confident it is often beneficial, although some physicians ridicule the practice as an *old woman's notion,* and say it intoxicates and inflames the blood. Every thing may be carried to excess; but it appears to me equally absurd to urge the intoxicating qualities of saffron, as an argument against the moderate and judicious use of it, as it would be to forbid the use of opium entirely, because it will occasion death when taken to excess. A few spoonsful of saffron tea, taken once or twice a-day, in all eruptive disorders, would greatly tend to prevent the retrocession of the eruption, from which such fatal effects so often arise, especially in very young children. I have always been in this practice, and never knew any eruption disappear till in its natural course it ought to do so, among all my children. Therefore, my fair readers, it is my sincere opinion, that you will do well, whenever your infants droop, and have highly feverish symptoms, to give them *a little saffron tea,* two or three times, and if the complaint is eruptive, it will assist nature in throwing it out; and no harm can result from it should it prove otherwise, as from long experience I am convinced, saffron, although a powerful stomachic, is perfectly harmless in its operation. A little snake root added to the saffron tea will often prove serviceable.

Small-Pox.

It is my sincere belief, and ardent hope, that the salutary practice of vaccine inoculation will, before the lapse of many ages, entirely exterminate this cruel disease. But as it is still prevalent in our southern states, and many a fond mother may be, at this moment, watching, with anxious fondness, the turn of the disorder in a beloved child; and similar instances may possibly occur in the northern and eastern parts of our country, where the disease is but little known, except by the dread it conveys, it may be proper to give such a description of the symptoms and method of cure as will enable parents to judge when they are visited by so unwelcome a guest, and to know how best to receive and expel him from their dwelling. We find the following description from the pen of Dr. Wallis.

" This complaint is occasioned by morbid matter of a peculiar nature absorbed into the habit from the external air, from contact of a person infected, or from inoculation, either by the inhaling vessels of the skin, lungs, membranes of the nose and mouth, or first passages, and has been divided, agreeably to the cuticular appearances, into distinct, confluent, coherent, or into common crystalline eruptions, full of thin serous matter; *verrucous*, resembling warts;

or *bloody*, filled with red fluid, or blood in a broken state.

" However, generally, now, we adhere to the terms *distinct* and *confluent;* but this seems of little use in practice; for they may be *distinct*, yet of a very bad kind; and *confluent*, yet very good; therefore, the more eligible division seems to be into *simple* and *malignant;* the first comprehending those which are the least, the last, those which are the most dangerous.

" *Causes.* The *remote* or *inducing* of this, as well as of every other species of infectious or contagious fever, is a predisposition or peculiarity of the constitution, to feel the impressions made by the morbid matter, productive of distress in the moving solids, and alteration of the fluids of the machine. The *proximate* or *immediate*, contaminating particles, peculiar to the small-pox, absorbed into the habit, and these producing febrile effects which vary according to the nature, or particular state of the constitution at that time.

" *Characteristic signs.* The only certain ones are the eruptions themselves, with their progressive concomitant symptoms, the appearance of which may be suspected in the first stage, if the attack should be sudden; if the small-pox should be the reigning epidemic, or the patient so situated that he has been thrown in the way of this specific infection; if pain should affect the back part of the head, fauces, loins, particularly the pit of the stomach, attended with vomiting, and that pain increased on pressure.

"*Cure.* The indications are, to diminish the assimilating or contaminating power of the morbid matter, and keep the fever within such bounds, that nature shall be enabled to separate from and throw out of the habit the offensive materials that cause the distress, which is done by so regulating the motions of the nervous and vascular systems, that the constitution may be put into a state to mitigate and support the succeeding contest with the greatest ease, and freedom from danger.

" And this knowledge we shall acquire, by considering the situation of the habit, the mode of living, and season of the year, with respect to the weather or constitution of the air, as these will dispose, more or less, to the production of inflammatory, nervous or putrescent febrile affections; for I am certain, that, according to the nature of the fever, so are we to regulate our conduct. Sometimes the disease is so extremely mild, that there is no need of medical assistance, though at the close, in order to clear the first passages from any foulness or offensive matter which may have been collected there during the progress of the complaint, it would be right to give two or three purges," which may be the same kind directed for the measles.

" At others, it is of a very dangerous nature, and requires the assistance and sagacity of no small share of medical knowledge, as it is accompanied with such a variety of threatening symptoms;" for which reason I have now extracted enough for our purpose, as no mother could think of trusting to her own skill in the management of this dreadful disease, when once convinced it was the small-pox. I can add very little from my own experience: although I have had the disorder myself, it was so very mild as scarcely to merit the name of disease, and all my children have been *vaccinated*. I, however, recollect perfectly well my attendants kept me almost frozen, and my diet for some weeks was very light, to which circumstances I probably owe the very favourable termination; for, being absent from my mother, the people who had the care of me, though otherwise very kind, trusted me to take my medicines, to which having a strong aversion, I threw them all away, which childish trick sufficiently proclaims I was then *a child*.

Chicken Pox.

This complaint is attended with no danger, although sometimes accompanied with a slight headach, great lassitude, and other feverish complaints, while the eruption is coming out and until it arrives at its height, which will be in the course of three or four days; at the commencement it will be proper to give a little saffron tea once a day. The eruption may be distinguished by the peculiar pellucid appearance of the pustules when they first rise; afterwards, those which do not get ruptured, gradually become white or yellowish, and resemble the *distinct* small-pox: no medicine is required, unless the feverish symptoms should run very high, which is rarely the case. Care must be taken to keep children who are ill with it, from the cold damps of the evening air, wetting their feet, &c. and to regulate their diet, letting it consist chiefly of light puddings, and broth and jellies; and, what is still better, bread and milk.

Dr. Wallis and other writers describe another species of this disease, which they denominate the *swine-pox*, which is much more virulent, but never fatal. Dr. Underwood gives a melancholy instance of the fatal effects of mistaking this for the small-pox.

Hooping-Cough.

This distressing disorder is known by the peculiar noise made in respiration during a fit of coughing, and which has given it its name. It usually begins with a dry, hard cough, which sometimes lasts many weeks before the *hooping* comes on. But I had better give the description from higher authority. It is thus learnedly described by Dr. Wallis.

"It is so called from the violence of the concussions, and that particular noise of *hooping* which is observable in the fits of coughing; also, *chincough,* from the dutch word *kincken,* to pant; in medical language, *tussis convulsiva* or *pertussis.*

"*Description.* In the beginning chiefly there is a dry cough, in which there is not thrown up any, or a very small quantity of thin serum, more or less acrid. Sometimes the cough is moist, and then a blackish or blue mucus, often extremely tenacious, is evacuated; at the same time, the extremities grow cold, the bowels are costive, and the blood is forced up copiously, and with great force, into the superior parts, breast and head: from whence, during the fit, the face grows turgid with blood, the veins swell, the arteries beat stronger and quicker, the eyes appear prominent, the tears flow, the eyelids puff up;

and sometimes the blood, particularly if a sneezing comes on, is forced out from the nostrils; sometimes the vessels of the lungs are ruptured, and there arises a spitting of blood; a hiccough often accompanies it, and very often vomiting. With respect to the convulsive affection, it does not appear generally till the second or third week from the attack; till that time it appears like a common cough, and then it comes on at different times of the day, and continues till some mucus is thrown up by the lungs, or the contents of the stomach evacuated, and then it ceases; when it has put on these appearances, its time of continuance is uncertain; it may go off in a few weeks, or remain some months. Before the fits come on there is some warning given, chiefly an uneasy sensation in breathing, and children will at this time catch hold of any thing that is near them, in order to support themselves during the fit of coughing, which they dread.

"*Cure.* The indications of which are, to correct or evacuate the peculiar infectious matter; to alleviate and lessen the violence and duration of the cough; and prevent those mischiefs which are likely to arise in the habit, or parts of it, from its excess. But as we know of no means either to correct or clear the constitution of the morbid matter creating the disease, we must, therefore, imitate Nature in her efforts, by such means as experience, founded on the knowledge of the laws of the animal economy, will point out to us, in accomplishing the two succeeding indications.

" In full habits, therefore, if the face swells much in coughing, looks red, and also the eyes, and other appearances of local plenitude show themselves, bleeding is essentially useful; and this must be repeated as long as such appearances render it necessary; but this must not be pushed too far; for then we should increase the convulsive affection; hence, in the slighter kinds of the disease it may be omitted; the body should be kept moderately open, not less than two or three stools procured every day; violent purging, for the reason above recited, might be hurtful. Gentle vomiting every day is beneficial in the forenoon, by small doses of antimonials, one or two spoonsful of the emetic mixture for a dose, or as much as will produce the effect; and should any feverish symptoms attend, a quarter or half a grain of tartarized antimony may be given at night with the powder, lessening or increasing the dose, according to the constitution; for this mode not only does good by the shock it gives to the habit, assisting expectoration, and clearing the stomach, but by determining the fluids to the surface, promoting perspiration, and keeping the body open, which last if it does not do, a little magnesia, or some other cooling purgative must be added; by persisting in this mode till evident symptoms of amendment presented themselves, then omitting the vomit to every second or third day; afterwards giving it once or twice a week, has been crowned with the desired success. Rubbing the pit of the stomach, and down the spine, with equal parts of rectified oil of amber, and spirits of wine, where there has been no inflammatory symptoms or febrile tendency; or after these had gone off, has been of great use; but bleeding and purgatives, when necessary, have preceded their use.

"However, in the general mode of management, I should, in the beginning, recommend vomiting and aperients, with bleeding, blistering, and use of antimonials, if necessary; small doses of cicuta; and where no febrile symptoms declared themselves, external antispasmodics. When the symptoms had considerably abated, tonics, particularly bark, should supply their place. And, in the *first period*, the diet should be abstemious and sparing, as in inflammatory fever if the symptoms ran high. In the *second*, the mode of living should be more generous; and should the lungs be affected by the violence of the disease, a course of ass's milk, riding, exercise, pure clear air, and the use of bark, would be proper. Indeed, in some cases, change of air is highly necessary, and very often alone produces the most salutary consequences. We must observe here, that often, when the coughing fit ceases, the patients are almost always perfectly relieved; but should they not, and the difficulty of breathing should continue, and there be any considerable febrile affections, *there is danger,* which must ever be suspected; for few die but under these circumstances; now and then bringing on immediate suffocation, and sometimes consumption; and often attended with extremely troublesome and painful affections; but it will sometimes occur in so mild a state, that all fear is unnecessary, and this will manifest itself by the gentleness of the symptoms; for though the complaint should be completely existing, accompanied with its certain symptoms of convulsive cough and hooping, if these should be moderate, and their returns observe distant periods; if the ejection of mucus from the lungs should be in no great degree, the difficulty of breathing, and febrile affections do not manifest themselves; and between the fits the patient preserves his usual habits of health, and the symptoms gradually decrease, Nature will be her own physician; in these cases little is necessary to be done."

I have here selected from a very learned and elaborate account of this afflicting complaint, such parts as I conceived adapted to domestic practice. Should children be dangerously ill, professional assistance will always be necessary, because every disease assumes different appearances in different constitutions; therefore, when attended with any degree of malignity, no general rule can be relied upon. All these variations Dr. Wallis particularizes, but no lady would trust her own judgment to discriminate, where her infant's life was at stake. What is here said is enough to enable us to know when more assistance is *requisite*, and this is absolutely necessary for every mother to know.

Several of my children have had it, and as the part of the country where we reside is remarkable for a pure, salubrious air, they were neither of them so ill as to be confined a moment, and took but little medicine. Elixir paregoric at night, and some expectorant drinks, such as hyssop tea, acidulated with lemon juice, or tamarinds, or cream of tartar, or linseed tea sweetened with double refined sugar, or honey, was all I found necessary for them; therefore, it would be my advice to all parents who reside in cities, and have it in their power, whenever their children are infected with the hooping cough, to remove them as far as possible from the place where the disease prevails, and permit them to use as much exercise as possible in a pure country air, free from the smoke and vapours of the town: this, in four instances out of five, would cause a mitigation of the most distressing symptoms. And although Dr. Wallis says nothing in favour of opiates in this disease, I must believe them of great service in allaying the spasmodic affections, as well as opening the chest, and assisting expectoration, especially the elixir paregoric; and that kind which has liquorice for an ingredient is to be preferred.

Inflammation of the Lungs.

This is a very distressing complaint, to which children from one to two years are very often subject. I have frequently known it brought on by violent exercise in a damp, cold air, and seen children who appeared only slightly affected with a cold at noon, come in from their play at night with a flushed face, violent headach, full hard pulse, breathing almost impeded, and attended by a wheezing noise extremely distressing, cough nearly incessant, and every symptom highly inflammatory, extending sometimes to a slight delirium. In these cases, I take the little patients to a warm room, give an emetic as soon as possible, bathe the feet and legs in warm water, and apply burdock leaves to the feet, if they are to be procured; if not, garlic drafts. I then put them to bed, and prevail upon them to drink freely of hyssop tea sweetened with honey. Should not the cough appear to abate after the operation of the emetic, in two or three hours I give a tea-spoonful, or less, according to the age of the child, of syrup of squills diluted with water, adding ten or fifteen drops of elixir paregoric; and in the morning exhibit a dose of senna and manna. If the child appears better in the morning, if the fever is abated, the breathing less difficult, and the cough somewhat relieved, a few days confinement, bathing the feet, and renewing the drafts every night, and giving a cup of hyssop tea every two or three hours, to promote expectoration and throw open the pores, will generally restore the little patient to health, with the addition of light and easy diet; but if the inflammatory symptoms increase rather than abate, the ensuing day, medical advice must be had, for this is an acute and often fatal complaint, if neglected; and if it does not readily yield to the little remedies here proposed, it would be wrong to trifle with it.

Ear-ach.

This may proceed from various causes; the most common are sudden cold affecting the part, either from exposing the head, uncovered, to the cold, after being very warm, or setting against a crack or crevice, so that a current of air shall strike directly upon the ear, which is a very delicate organ, easily subject to inflammation, which often ends in deafness, or perpetual ulcers, which are extremely afflicting and troublesome.

The ear-ach, also, sometimes proceeds from hardened wax sticking in the ear, or worms being bred there, from eggs laid in the wax by the flesh fly, which Dr. Wallis mentions as being sometimes the case. It is, also, spasmodic, and is then often very severe, and likely to recur frequently, being occasioned by every little cold. Dr. Underwood, recommends the juice of rue, and two or three drops of laudanum, when this is the cause; or six or eight drops of laudanum, made warm, and dropped into the ear with a marrow spoon. But the worst disorder of the ear is an abscess forming within it, which is often occasioned by a sudden cold, but is more frequently owing to the translation of morbid matter to the ear, usually at the crisis of some malignant fever, or those of the typhus kind; and these ulcers are very difficult to heal, often continuing to discharge many months, and sometimes are never perfectly healed, but occasion deafness, and all its unpleasant effects; and when they are actually healed, the part continues subject to them, upon the slightest cold. When this happens there is no relief until a suppuration takes place, to which end we must bend all our endeavours. Roasted onions are exceedingly good applied warm to the part; the heart of the onion should be wrapped in fine lawn, and inserted into the cavity of the ear, and the remainder put into a fine linen or lawn bag, and applied as close as possible, so as to exclude the cold air; these should be changed as often as they become cold or dry. If the pain continues violent, and the onions fail to give ease, chamomile flowers boiled in water, so as to form a very strong decoction, and then the flowers put into two little flannel bags, and dipped alternately into the decoction, kept hot for the purpose, and applied to the ear, and changed as often as they grow cool, will often give great relief; but no lasting ease can be expected until the abscess breaks, which is usually preceded by excruciating pain, and succeeded by perfect ease, excepting the extreme soreness, which often continues several days, as will the discharge not unfrequently a fortnight. When the abscess breaks, the ear should be syringed out perfectly clean every day, with warm Castile soap suds, afterwards injecting into it tincture of myrrh diluted with water, or a weak solution of sugar of lead, and stopping the orifice with a little lint or wool, to keep out the cold. Dr. Underwood gives the following directions, when the discharge becomes fetid and of long standing.

" It is not uncommon to meet with fetid discharges from the internal ear, either with or without inflammation and external soreness; but this is usually in children of one or more years old, rather than very young infants. If a little cooling physic, and wiping out the matter frequently, does not remove the complaint, cleansing injections should be used, and the following warm acoustic dropped into the ear: Take oil of almonds, half an ounce; rectified oil of amber, twenty drops; camphorated spirits, half a drachm; tincture of castor, one drachm; mix these together, and instil four or six drops, previously made warm, into the ear affected, night and morning, afterwards inserting loosely a bit of cotton to prevent the escape of the oil. The child should also be made to lie as much as may be on the affected side, that the discharge may have a free vent. Should the quantity and fetid smell of the matter increase, a blister should be kept on the nape of the neck, a few purges of calomel be taken, and, on the intermediate days, very small doses of the powder of quicksilver with sulphur, as kept in the shops. But above all, fumigations with the red sulphurated quicksilver, and quicksilver with sulphur mixed together, should be made use of morning and evening, from which I have seen the very best effects; when the discharge and fetid smell have been very great, and the ulcer of long standing. To this end, a tube or funnel must be properly adapted."

Scald Head.

There is little danger of this complaint occurring among children, who are properly attended to; little else being necessary to prevent it than perfect cleanliness, and combing the head every day with a fine comb; it is, however, sometimes the consequence of a bad habit of body, and is united with scrophula, and when this is the case, it is often difficult to cure. It is said to be contagious, and frequently communicated at school. If this is the case, every child must be exposed to it who attends a public seminary, and, therefore, it may be desirable to know the best mode of management. Dr. Underwood gives the following:

"From some considerable experience, I may venture to say, that being usually a mere complaint of the skin, it may be most successfully treated by external applications. This disease is seated in the little glands at the roots of the hair, is sometimes dry but at others moist, and then produces little ulcers; which being thoroughly cleansed, and made to digest, may be safely healed up; as I have found in many other affections of the skin, in which the system has often over scrupulously been conceived to be concerned. It is not uncommon, I know, to administer a variety of internal remedies, and perhaps they may sometimes be required; though I think I have seldom given any thing more than lime water, or a decoction of the woods, and a few purges at the decline of the eruption.

" If the complaint be taken early, before it has spread far over the head, and while the scabby patches are small and distinct, it may frequently be cured by an ointment made of equal parts of sulphur, flour of mustard, and powder of staves-acre, mixed up with lard or butter, or with the sulphur ointment, with a small addition of the white calx of mercury. And this last preparation may very safely be made use of, if the patient be kept within doors and the body properly open; as it will be necessary to rub

U

in only a small portion once or twice a day, on the parts immediately affected. But if the disease should spread, or has already extended itself over a great part of the head, the hair must be shaved off, and the head washed twice a day with a strong decoction of tobacco; repeating this process until the scabs disappear, and the hair grows up from the parts they had occupied. Or, instead of the decoction of tobacco, the head may be well washed with the soap lotion of the shops, with the addition of a small quantity of the pure water of kali; and the scabs anointed with the ointment of nitrated quicksilver, in place of the sulphur ointment and calx of mercury; the former being a very powerful as well as safe application, and may be used in any quantity that may be necessary.

" But the complaint is sometimes of long standing before medical assistance is solicited, and is not only extended over the whole head, but the scabs are thick, and return as often as they may fall off. I have, however, never failed to cure common scald head by a method not so much, generally, unknown, as too seldom complied with in time, on account of its supposed severity. It consists only in well washing the head, first shaved, with a piece of flannel and a strong lather of soap suds, and then rubbing in very forcibly the tar ointment, and a good quantity of the powder of white hellebore, for near an hour at a time, always using it very warm; and covering the head with a bladder to preserve the ointment on the part, as well as to prevent it from sticking to the cap, or other covering made use of. When this has been done three or four times, not only the scabs but the hairs will also loosen, which must be pulled out, however unpleasant the operation may be, as it will, indeed, prove a kindness in the end; and must be repeated until all the hairs be taken out; after which new hair will rise free from scabs, which is a sufficient indication that the disorder is effectually removed."

Herpes or Ringworm.

" The ringworm, like the foregoing complaint, is a disease of the skin, infesting some children almost annually, and appearing in dry scurfy blotches on different parts of the body. It becomes troublesome chiefly from the violent itching that constantly attends it, and would probably get well of itself: it even, sometimes, has the appearance of being critical; or is, perhaps, rather an indication of some favourable change in valetudinarians, especially in adults; who are, sometimes, found getting the better of lingering complaints at the time the ringworm makes its appearance. It is, however, often a blemish, as it frequently attacks the hands and face, especially the forehead.

" 'The ringworm is certainly very easily cured, the eruption yielding very readily to stimulating and astringent remedies. Ink, therefore, (as it contains an infusion of galls,) has been a common, though inelegant application, and may serve very well where better forms are not at hand. It is sometimes made into a paste, with flower of mustard. Spirits of wine, lotions of diluted extract of lead, with the addition of vinegar, or white vitriol; and ointments containing lead, answer very well: but the ointment of nitrated quicksilver is preferable to most others.

"The use of the flesh brush is a good preventive in habits accustomed to the complaint. It can be only in unhealthy children, that there can be any fear in regard to external applications, or need of internal remedies. Should the ringworm spread, and become sore, it should be treated as directed below."

The Ulcerating Herpes.

"This is a malignant species of the above complaint, but is generally local; it is mentioned in this place, as having relation to the former; being itself rather a sore than an eruption, and not very common in children. Suppurative, or digestive applications may be made use of in the early stage of the complaint, such as ointments of minium, soap, and Venice turpentine, or a suppurative poultice, made of figs, onions, and white lily roots, boiled in water to a soft pulp, with or without the addition of a little bread and milk; in order to liberate the deceased and obstructed glands on the surface, and absorb the acrid discharge. After this, the parts should be washed with some soap lotion; and lastly, with a strong solution of vitriol. Should these fail, the ointment of nitrated quicksilver will be proper; and, as the last remedy, caustic applications, of which butter of antimony is the best, with which the little ulcers may be touched lightly, from time to time, under the eye of some medical person. The patient may also take a decoction of burdock roots, or sarsaparilla."

The Shingles.

" THE shingles is a complaint different from the foregoing, but being rarely met with, has not been accurately distinguished from other herpetic eruptions. It appears in the form of blisters, of different sizes, with or without some redness between them. This, however, is an affection of the system, which the others are not, and is attended with fever, as well as often preceded by shivering, sickness, and sometimes even vomiting, but is not dangerous.

" The feverish symptoms, however, do not wholly disappear on the eruption of the pustules; which gradually subsides as the fluid they contain acquires a thicker consistence; after which the pustules dry off in the form of dark-coloured crusts; and the disease terminates in the period of from eight to ten days, and not unfrequently without medical aid. But in the confluent species, which is attended with the most fever, the patient should be kept in a warm atmosphere, take some light cordial," (such as saffron tea,) " and when the pustules are drying off, a gentle purgative should be administered. It is among the vulgar errors, I believe, that when this complaint appears on the breast or loins, if it should extend round the whole body it would prove fatal. This form of the disease is termed the herpetic belt."

One of my children was attacked by this complaint a few months past. It made its appearance rather upon the left side of his body, in the form of a cluster of little blisters with a very inflamed base, and was extremely sore to the touch; it gradually spread over his bowels the length of three or four inches, and there appeared an evident inflammation extending from the part affected up to his arm-pit, where he complained of pain; he had been drooping for several days before I discovered the eruption, and complained much of sickness at his stomach, and headach, which symptoms continued until the eruption began to dry off. The physician to whom I applied, directed a solution of sugar of lead, in vinegar and water. I applied cloths, wet in this liquid, warm, to the part several times a day, which cooled the inflammation, and gave him great relief. I let him drink several times a little saffron tea, to defend his stomach, and after the pustules began to dry off, I gave him elderberry syrup several times, which proved gently purgative, and soon restored him to his wonted health.

Canker in the Mouth.

Children who cut their teeth painfully are very subject to this complaint, which must greatly aggravate their distress. I have found great relief from the root of the *wake-robin*, or *dragon root*, as it is termed in this country, grated and mixed with honey, and used in the manner borax is prescribed for the thrush, in the former part of this work; about a teaspoonful of the fresh root mixed with three table spoonsful of honey, or if the root is dry, a larger proportion must be used; this mixture put upon the child's tongue, or touched about the lips several times a day, will frequently perform a cure. **Dr. Underwood** esteems it a very slight complaint; but I have known infants very ill with it, and totally unable to eat or suck for several days, except a little milk from a spoon, and that with great pain; and when we reflect upon the very great inconvenience and distress we feel from ever so small a speck upon the mouth or tongue, we may judge of the tortures the poor little creatures must endure who have their whole mouth and throat lined with ulcers, as is often the case. A very good gargle may be made by simmering a little saffron, sage, gold thread, and a very small bunch of sumack berries in simple water, and making it very sweet with honey, and dusting in a little burnt alum; this cannot be used, however, to advantage for very young children, because we cannot instruct them to gargle the mouth sufficiently in a proper manner; nevertheless, should the dragon root and honey fail of the desired effect, this decoction may be put occasionally into the mouth, as no harm can result from their swallowing it in small quantities at a time; and if the canker extends into the throat, it may be necessary. Small doses of calomel mixed with honey, and given once or twice a week, I have found serviceable in this complaint among my children; and after the scales begin to fall off, and the mouth is in some measure healed, magnesia should be given several times, to absorb and assist in discharging the acrimony lodged in the stomach and bowels, during this disagreeable complaint. But magnesia is so apt to stick about the mouth and throat, that it is almost cruel to force it down while they are very sore. If a gentle purgative is thought necessary, syrup of violets, or elder berries, or each alternately, will be found very salutary, especially the latter.

Chilblains.

THIS troublesome complaint may be entirely prevented by keeping the feet and hands covered from the cold; but should it occur, as it frequently will in our inclement climate, however careful we may be, it may generally be removed by bathing the feet in warm water, and then rubbing them well with opedeldoc, either the liquid opedeldoc, or that known by the name of Sears's opedeldoc, will answer, the qualities being essentially the same. The part must then be kept from extreme cold, until perfectly recovered. But if the complaint has proceeded to suppuration, as it often will, after the above applications, the thin skin from off the hog's suet, or, when that cannot be had, the veal caul should be applied to the part, and secured with linen bandages, to prevent the stockings fretting it: this mode will seldom fail of removing the complaint, if persevered in, and *began* in due season; but if the disorder is slighted, or neglected entirely, it often proves troublesome through life.

Warts.

THE green bark of the sweet elder bush is a sovereign remedy for warts, which are important rather as a deformity than a disease. They will, however, sometimes become inflamed and sore; in which case, the above application never fails to cure, if it can be obtained;

but as this is difficult for those that reside in cities, other remedies therefore may be tried; among which, ligatures of horse hair or silk, are strongly recommended, as being the most effectual method of destroying the excrescence; but I have seen them cured in a short time, when the hands were almost covered with them, by being rubbed for some minutes every day with a piece of gold or silver.

Stithe or Stye.

The stithe is a small inflamed tumour on the edge of the eyelid, more commonly on the side towards the nose; but there are sometimes two or more at a time. " It is occasioned by an obstruction in the glands of the eyelids, and the matter being enclosed in a hard cist or bag, the inflammation often returns in the same spot, till the cist being destroyed by repeated suppurations, the cavity is afterwards filled up, and the complaint disappears. All that is necessary to prevent the return of this temporary blemish, is, to imitate this process of nature. To this end the little abscess, as soon as it breaks, should be lightly touched with the caustic, called nitrated silver, cut to a point, (cautiously avoiding doing injury to the eye,) which, by destroying the cist, at once removes the complaint."

Underwood.

CHAPTER V.

SECTION I.

A brief Description of such Plants, and their respective Medicinal Qualities, as are mentioned in the preceding pages; with many others, peculiarly serviceable in the Complaints of Children.

> " Life's lowest, but far greatest sphere I sing,
> " Of all things that adorn the gaudy spring;
> " Such as in deserts live, whom, unconfined,
> " None but the simple laws of Nature bind;
> " And those who, growing tame by human care,
> " The well-bred citizens of gardens are;
> " Those that aspire to Sol their sire's bright face,
> " Or stoop into their mother Earth's embrace;
> " Such as drink streams, or wells, or those, dry fed,
> " Who have Jove only for their Ganymede;
> " And all that Solomon's lost work of old
> " (Ah! fatal loss!) so wisely did unfold.
> " Though I the oak's vivacious age should live,
> " I ne'er to all their names in verse could give."
>
> COWLEY.

THE beneficent creator has enriched our country with many simples calculated to relieve the diseases incident to our climate, and if resorted to in season would often supersede the use of compounded drugs, especially in the disorders peculiar to childhood: therefore, every mother ought to have a general knowledge of them, so that she may prescribe for slight complaints with ease to herself, and infinite benefit to her little family.

To assist her in obtaining this knowledge, I have collected a brief history of the plants in most esteem, that, by having them all under her eye, she may readily choose those adapted to the present complaints of her children; and as I shall take my description of their virtues from the most approved medical books, where my own experimental knowledge fails, my readers may rely upon the directions given, that they are so far correct, as no danger can arise from following them implicitly.

Arum or Wake Robin.

COMMONLY known in this country by the names of dragon root, and wild turnip. It grows wild in all parts of New-England, and is in great repute for its medicinal virtues. In March or April, it sends forth two branches from one stalk, and between them arises a purple pistil, enclosed in a sheath beautifully striped with purple and white, which curls over the pistil as it grows towards maturity; till at length, this is succeeded, in July and August, by a bunch of red berries. All parts of the plant are very pungent; but when fresh, the root resembles the common turnip in appearance, and children have been frequently deluded by it, and induced to taste it to their sorrow; for while fresh, it is almost intolerable, so very acrimonious is the juice; but after it is dry, it loses much of this quality, and in this form it is chiefly used in this country, in domestic practice, and is excellent in colds and colics, for the canker, and windy complaints in infants. The fresh root is highly recommended in the Edinburgh Dispensatory.

" The root is a powerful stimulant. It is reckoned a medicine of great efficacy in some cachectic and chlorotic cases, in weakness of the stomach occasioned by a load of viscid phlegm. Great benefit has been obtained from it in rheumatic pains, particularly those of the fixed kind, and which were deep seated. In those cases, from ten grains to a scruple of the fresh root may be given twice or thrice a day, made into a bolus or emulsion with unctuous and mucilaginous substances, which cover its pungency, and prevent its making any painful impression on the tongue. It generally excites a slight tingling sensation through the whole habit; and when the patient is kept warm in bed, produces a copious sweat." The root may be gathered any time in the year, as it is said to be equally good at all times. It loses its virtue if kept too long, and becomes perfectly insipid to the taste.

Alder.

The leaves and bark of the alder tree have a bitter, stiptic, disagreeable taste. The bark is recommended in intermittent fevers, and a decoction of it in gargarisms for inflammations of the tonsils.

Edinburgh Dispensatory.

Ash Tree.

There are several kinds of ash in this country, adorning our forests in great abundance. The sap of the black and white ash is said to be an excellent remedy for the earach; and if the use of it is continued for a length of time after the breaking of an abscess within the ear, it will prevent a return of the complaint. It is obtained by placing a stick of the wood green from the forest across the andirons, at a convenient distance from the fire, so that the middle part may burn gently; the sap will ooze out at each end, and must be received into cups placed for the purpose, then strained and put into a phial for use; when used it should be made warm and injected into the ear with a syringe, or, when that cannot be had, carefully dropped in with a tea-spoon, and a piece of lint or cotton inserted to keep out the cold air. This sap is used by the aborigines of our country, in the cure of cancers, and frequently with great success; they prescribe it internally and externally. The bark and watery extract is good in intermittent fevers. The bark of another species called *prickly ash,* steeped in brandy, is highly recommended in rheumatic complaints.

Anise Seed.

THE plant producing these seeds may be cultivated in our gardens. They are carminative, and moderately anodyne: the essential oil is an ingredient in the paregoric elixir, and is used by itself dropped on sugar in doses of from two to twenty drops in disorders of the breast, and spasmodic windy complaints, so afflicting to infants. The seed in infusion or powder are said to be preferable in flatulent colics.

Angelica.

This finely aromatic plant grows wild in the woods and fields in Vermont, and many if not all the other states. It is frequently preserved, and forms an elegant confection, and is of use as a carminative; children who have flatulent complaints will readily take it in this form. The root is an ingredient in the aromatic tincture of the shops.

Avens Root.

This plant, or rather the root of it, was highly esteemed by the natives of this country, and they have transmitted its honours unimpaired to their successors in the soil. The common people esteem it almost a specific in many cases, and many of them use it in their houses instead of coffee, or chocolate, the last of which, a decoction of it greatly resembles. The taste is not unpleasant, and children who are out of health would reap great benefit from taking it for their breakfast and supper, which they would readily do, if deceived with the addition of cream and sugar. It is highly recommended in the Edinburgh Dispensatory as a powerful stomachic, and for strengthening the tone of the viscera in general. The root has a warm astringent taste, and a pleasant aromatic smell, especially in the spring. It yields on distillation an elegant odoriferous essential oil, which concretes into a flaky form.

Agrimony.

This plant grows wild in the fields and highways, and has an acrid rough taste, somewhat aromatic. A tea of it is often serviceable in fevers, especially those of the dysenteric kind. Digested in whey it affords a diet-drink, grateful to the palate and stomach.

Bayberry Bush.

This valuable bush grows wild in many parts of America. The leaves and berries are in great repute for their warm carminative qualities. Dr. Motherby thinks them highly stomachic. The berries yield on distillation a considerable quantity of aromatic essential oil, which is beneficial in flatulent colics, dropped on sugar, from two to ten and fifteen drops for a dose. They also yield on pressure an insipid oil, which, when boiled, cools into the consistence of wax, of a yellowish green colour; but the more common mode of obtaining this oil is, by boiling the berries a considerable time in fair water, then setting the vessel by to cool; the berries will subside to the bottom, and the wax cool on the top; it must then be taken off, and melted again by itself, in a clean earthen vessel, or a copper, that is well tinned upon the inside; when melted, it must be strained through a thin strainer, or fine sieve, into proper moulds, to form it into cakes. This wax has an agreeable smell, and has long been regarded as an excellent medicine in the dysentery. It may be grated and mixed with loaf sugar, and children will take it very readily; they should take it several times a day, to be of any service. It is likewise used in ointments, for burns, and other complaints. In addition to all these virtues, it will make candles equal in hardness to spermaceti, and superior in fragrance. It is frequently used to impart an agreeable perfume to common household candles.

Balsam of Fir.

This elegant balsam is procured from an evergreen tree, a native of the northern parts of the United States, and of Canada, from whence it is styled in the Dispensatory, *Canada balsam.* It is, however, a common forest tree, and the balsam is procured from little globules on the trunk of the tree, and exudes upon pricking them, when it should be received into phials, and stopped close, as the air dries it, and renders it glutinous. This balsam is perfectly pellucid, and is said to possess all the virtues of the balsam copaiva. It is esteemed in domestic practice, in the neighbourhood where it grows, as almost a specific for green wounds and inward bruises.

Baum or Balm.

THIS well known and excellent herb needs no particular description; it is usually cultivated in our gardens, and is divided into two species, the *high* and the *low* baum; the low baum is in the highest esteem, generally, and is undoubtedly very excellent in infusion for dry, parching fevers; the tea, acidulated with lemon juice, or cream of tartar, should always form a variety, at least, in the diluting drinks, in all feverish complaints.

Y

Blood Root.

This is a very valuable simple. It grows wild in the woods in New England. The juice of the fresh root resembles blood in the colour; the roots themselves look very much like small red beets; I have never seen any larger than a man's finger. It is a very strong pungent bitter. Rectified spirits extracts all its virtues, and a tincture of it is frequently used in domestic practice for the jaundice, weakness of the stomach, and many other complaints. It is a powerful styptic, peculiarly excellent for bleeding at the lungs, or stomach. It is also ascertained to be of great service to children who are subject to biles, and other purulent humours; for this purpose, the roots are cut in thin slices and toasted in the manner coffee is done; when perfectly brown, it must be put into a bottle, and equal quantities of rectified spirit and water added to it; after it has infused several days, a teaspoonful in a little water may be given a child of one or two years twice a day, until it has the desired effect; and if the child is older, the quantity may be increased to a table-spoonful for a dose. When fresh, the root is both emetic and cathartic; toasting deprives it of those qualities in a great degree. I think it merits the attention of gentlemen of the faculty.

Burdock.

This is a well known plant, but its medicinal virtues are not duly estimated. It is said to be excellent in removing every obstruction. A table-spoonful of the seed, bruised and taken in a little water, or any other menstrua, will often afford great relief in the ague in the face. I have repeatedly had occasion in the foregoing pages to recommend the leaves, as drafts in all febrile affections, which I now beg leave to enforce. Many people dry the leaves, and preserve them for this purpose, and when wanted, boil them in vinegar and water, and apply them warm to the feet; there should be barely liquor enough to moisten the leaves.

Carua or Caraway Seeds.

THESE seeds are so well known, and universally admired, for culinary purposes, I shall only observe that the essential oil, and simple distilled water, are the best cordial and carminative medicines I have ever used for infants.

Elder.

THERE are several species of this plant. That which puts forth large umbelliferous bunches of white flowers in June, followed in August and September, by black berries, growing in the same form, and generally known by the name of sweet elder, is the sort in most esteem for medicinal uses. The young buds and shoots are said to be so powerfully purgative as to be unsafe; the inner green bark is gently laxative, and excellent in ointments for all kinds of hot painful eruptions. It is made by simmering the green bark in oil or lard, until they become of a green colour. An infusion of the flowers is an excellent purgative for very young infants, and is said to effectually cure the St. Anthony's Fire, or Eresipelas, if drank very freely for some time. The berries may be dried, and in that form kept for use; a table-spoonful of them steeped in a gill of water, until half evaporated, and sweetened with honey, or syrup of roses, or even coarse sugar, will prove powerfully cathartic for infants and young children. The expressed juice formed into a syrup, with an equal quantity of honey, or treacle, will keep many months, and is excellent for children who are affected with cutaneous eruptions. It must be given in doses of from one to two table-spoonsful every morning, for several days, to have the desired effect in those cases; but as a laxative in cases of constipation, a table-spoonful to an infant, from four months to a year will produce the end required. To an older child the dose must be increased.

Elecampane.

This is a large downy plant, growing wild in all our woods and fields. It is said to expel poison, by causing perspiration. The root when dry has an agreeable smell; its taste is glutinous and somewhat of an aromatic bitter; when nicely candied it forms an elegant confection, highly recommended for humoral coughs and asthmas, as a stomachic, and for strengthening the system in general. Children, who are subject to coughs, may receive great benefit from it in this form, and they are usually fond of it.

Sweet, or Slippery Elm.

This is a forest tree, very common in America. The inner bark is in great repute in cutaneous eruptions, and is taken in decoction, and spirituous infusion. In the Edinburgh Dispensatory, we find this short notice: "This bark has a mild astringent taste; a decoction formed from it, by boiling an ounce in a pound of water, to the consumption of one half, has been highly recommended by some, particularly by Dr. Letsome, in obstinate cutaneous disorders." A cataplasm formed by boiling this bark, previously bruised, in milk and water until it becomes perfectly soft and mucilaginous, is one of the best applications for a bile, or painful tumour, I ever tried in my family. It is extremely easy and grateful.

Sweet Fennel.

It is an old adage that "he who *sows fennel, sows sorrow.*" How this poor plant came to be loaded with such a stigma it would be difficult to say; however, when we reflect that whether we sow fennel or not, sorrow will spring up in all our paths, it is needless to banish this very excellent herb, lest it should come accompanied by its meagre companion; therefore, let us cultivate it for its known virtues, which are many. It is said the seeds are good in the small-pox, measles, malignant fevers, heaviness, headachs, indigestion, flatulent colics, and many other complaints, from whence it might seem, that "*he who sows fennel might banish sorrow.*" The dose of the seeds is from half a drachm to a drachm; of the essential oil, from two to twenty drops, on sugar.

Fever Bush.

This is a beautiful fragrant shrub, growing wild in many parts of America, and in high repute among the inhabitants as a febrifuge, from whence its name. The whole plant is highly aromatic; the bark chewed a short time has much the taste of lemon peel, though less pungent. A tea made from any part of the bush is both aromatic and mucilaginous, and is found very efficacious in dysenteries. It will, probably, one day or other, attract the attention of the medical societies in this country, or has already done so.

Sweet Flagroot.

This is an elegant aromatic, and is found in abundance in low marshy grounds. It is a powerful carminative for infants, and is said to prove stimulating to people of all ages, occasioning agreeable sensations in the mind. The candied root is sufficiently agreeable, and highly esteemed as an antiseptic, and used to prevent contagion when epidemic diseases are prevalent.

Gold Thread.

This is a small vine which runs on the ground in moist woody lands in America. The root, which is the part used for medicinal purposes, spreads itself just below the surface of the earth, from whence it is easily drawn by handsful, and resembles a large entangled skein of thread of a bright gold colour, from whence it derives its name. It is a fine astringent bitter. The Indians use it for canker in the mouth, and our physicians find it an excellent remedy in gargarisms for that complaint.

House Leek.

THIS is a singular plant, which loves to cling to old stumps and hedges; it looks, while growing, like a cluster of green balls, but upon nearer inspection, they assume the form of roses; the leaves are thick, and appear full of a mucilaginous juice; simmered in fresh butter, oil, or lard, it makes an excellent ointment for burns, or any cutaneous eruptions. There is another species also, called *air plant*, which is very beautiful, and has nearly the same virtues.

Hyssop.

THIS is an invaluable herb among children, especially those who are liable to have lung complaints. In inflammatory fevers, it has not its superior. A very strong decoction of it, sweetened with honey, and a small piece of spermaceti dissolved in it, taken in doses of a table-spoonful several times a day, repeatedly cured one of my children who was very subject to inflammation on the lungs, and has finally conquered the disease.

Catmint or Catnip.

This is an excellent herb for infants. The distilled water and essential oil, are powerful in their bowel complaints. It is said to partake of the virtues of mint and penny-royal. It grows in great abundance in fields and hedges, and is too well known to need a particular description. I have distilled it in the flower, and found it yield a small quantity of very pungent essential oil, which cooled in white flakes, but readily dissolved in rectified spirit. I also distilled it when the seeds were just formed, and obtained a very clear essential oil of a dark green colour, resembling the other in smell and flavour.

Spearmint.

THIS plant is one of the most powerful vermifuges we have in our vegetable kingdom, and is found in all our highways. It yields a large quantity of very limpid essential oil, which dropped on sugar in doses of from one to six drops, and given to children who are subject to worms, every morning for a length of time, will frequently expel numbers of those vermin, and remove many disagreeable symptoms occasioned by them. The distilled water is highly stomachic; the leaves, when fresh or dry, drank as a tea, is not less efficacious, though not quite so convenient. " Their virtues are those of a warm stomachic and carminative. In loss of appetite, nausea, continual retchings to vomit, and, as Boerhaave expresses it, in almost paralytic weaknesses of the stomach, few simples are, perhaps, of equal efficacy."

Edinburgh Dispensatory.

Tansy.

This herb is a warm deobstruent bitter, and an excellent vermifuge for children. The essential oil, or essence, may be given in the same manner as the last-mentioned plants.

Peppermint.

The essence procured from this plant, has long maintained a conspicuous place in public opinion; but, although more agreeable, it is, perhaps, inferior in some respects to the spearmint. It is, however, an excellent medicine in many cases, especially faintness and loss of appetite. It grows in abundance in almost every garden, but is not a native of our soil,

z

Pennyroyal.

Is a native, and one of our choicest plants. " Pennyroyal is a warm pungent herb, of the aromatic kind, similar to mint, but more acrid and less agreeable. It has long been held in great esteem, as an aperient and deobstruent, particularly in hysteric complaints; for this purpose, the distilled water is generally used, or an infusion of the leaves."

Edinburgh Dispensatory.

Sassafras.

This is an American tree of the laurel kind. The bark of the root, and, indeed, of the whole tree, is very aromatic; not unlike mace in its taste, and was used in the late American war as spice, by many highly patriotic people. " As to the virtues of sassafras, it is a warm aperient and corroborant, and frequently employed with good success, for purifying the blood and juices; for these purposes an infusion made from the rasped root or bark, may be used as tea. Sassafras yields an extremely fragrant essential oil, of a penetrating pungent taste, so ponderous, notwithstanding the lightness of the drug itself, as to sink in water."

Edinburgh Dispensatory.

Sumach.

THE wood of this tree, which grows wild in every part of the United States, is a very beautiful bright yellow, and has been made into snuff boxes, and other toys, and sent to Europe, by way of curiosity. The leaves, berries, and seeds, have an acid astringent taste, and are very efficacious, in gargles, for the canker, and inflammations of the tonsils. The bark of the root bruised and boiled in milk and water, and a little Indian meal stirred into it, while cooling, makes an excellent application for burns, and is said to prevent an eschar.

Thorough Wort or Stanch Blood.

THE names of this herb are highly indicative of its qualities. It is an umbelliferous plant, and is remarkable for the stock appearing to grow through the leaves. I don't find it in the Edinburgh Dispensatory, and am not scientific enough to give a technical account of its properties. However, it grows wild in most parts of New-England, and is in great esteem among the inhabitants, as an emetic and cathartic. It frequently gives relief in bilious colics, when all other medicines are ejected, or fail of the desired effect. It has a bitter astringent taste, and is a well known styptic. It will stop the bleeding of fresh wounds, for which purpose the leaves may be applied green, or powdered on when dry. But its superior excellence lies in its efficacy in curing internal hæmorrhages. Drinking a pint of tea made from this plant, every night for twelve months, cured my father of a dangerous bleeding at the stomach, which had baffled the physician's skill for seven years, and he appeared fast sinking to his grave. After this, he lived many years in perfect health.

Strawberry Bush.

THE well known and delicious fruit, the product of this bush or plant, it may seem, renders it so well known as not to require any further description; but although as a dessert it is known, its medicinal virtues are not so well understood. Many, perhaps, are to be told, that the plant taken in infusion as a tea, is excellent for the jaundice; that the leaves bruised and applied to a fresh wound, will stop bleeding; and what will be more interesting to the ladies, the fruit is said to dissolve tartareous incrustations of the teeth. Surely so elegant a dentifrice cannot easily be formed by art. The fruit is also said to be peculiarly efficacious in curing long and obstinate diarrhœas, and an excellent remedy for the scurvy.

Violets.

> " (Io triumph!) now, now the Spring comes on,
> " In solemn state and high procession,
> " Whilst I, the beauteous Violet, before him go,
> " And usher in the gaudy show.
> " As it becomes the child of such a sire,
> " I'm wrapt in purple; the first born of Spring,
> " The marks of my legitimation bring,
> " And all the tokens of his verdant empire wear.
> " Clad like a princely babe, and born in state,
> " I all your regal titles hate,
> " Nor priding in my blood, and mighty birth,
> " Unnatural plant, despise the lap of mother Earth."
>
> COWLEY.

IN April, these lovely little flowers adorn our fields in great abundance; perfuming the air, as if commissioned by a bountiful Parent to regale and delight his vast family, after the tedious lapse of ungenial winter, and seem designed by nature for a medicine for her infant offspring, at this season, when the blood requires something laxative and aperient, for which purpose there is nothing superior to a *syrup of violets*. It is thus prepared: "Take of fresh violets, one pound; boiling water, two quarts; double refined sugar, seven pounds and a half; macerate the flowers in the water twenty-four hours, in a glass, or glazed earthen vessel; then strain, and to the strained liquor, add the sugar powdered, and make into a syrup; a table spoonful or two proves gently laxative to children."

Edinburgh Dispensatory

CHAPTER VI.

CONCLUSION.

"But trust me, when you have done all this,
"Much will be missing still, and much will be amiss."

MILTON'S ODES.

I HAVE thus, to the best of my abilities, fulfilled my promise, and endeavoured to enable my fair readers to nurse their lovely offspring *from the birth until two years old,* or till they arrive at an age requiring *comparatively* less attention. And if my plan is adopted, I flatter myself, they will acquire such a stock of health and strength by that time, as with only common care through the remainder of their childhood, will ensure their exemption from the various complaints, arising from debility, weakness of body, and relaxation of the nervous system, such as convulsions, epilepsies, fevers, consumptions, king's evil, rickets, and many others, too numerous to mention; and which, for want of proper attention to their first complaints, and sufficient exercise in the open air, too frequently afflict them through a long life, or sink them to an early grave. Therefore, let me once more entreat for my young friends who have arrived at an age when nature prompts them to seek health and happiness in sportive gambols suited to their age, that they may not be confined to the house, to their infinite vexation, and the imminent danger of undoing all you have hitherto done. Surely it is wrong to immure *boys*, from a desire to see them look fair and delicate, whose chief attraction, both now and in after life, must consist in their courage, strength, and activity. To say nothing of our duty, as *citizens*, while forming the future guardians of our beloved country, it is undoubtedly our duty, as *mothers*, to bring up our sons in such a manner as shall render them most useful and happy; and one of the most effectual steps towards this desirable end, is to let them have the free use of their limbs during this active period of their lives, and restricting them to the most simple and nutritious diet—

> ———" By arts like these,
> " Laconia nursed of old her hardy sons,
> " And Rome's unconquer'd legions urged their way,
> " Unhurt, through every toil, in every clime."
>
> ARMSTRONG.

And even our lovely and interesting daughters will be more lovely and more interesting, if adorned with the roses of health, entwined with the lilies of innocence and delicacy. And this is the time to strengthen their constitutions, and give grace and activity to their limbs, by frequent unrestrained exercise in the open air. Now, before female vanity begins to operate, and teaches them to shun the light kisses of the passing zephyr, lest they should leave the unseemly traces of the rude salute on the damask cheek, or lily neck: now, while the infant heart, elate with joy and unconscious of remark, bounds with delight at every change of scene, eagerly springing from object to object, ever seeking and ever finding new and innocent enjoyments, while indulgent Nature seems to say—

> " For *thee* my borders nurse the fragrant wreath,
> " My fountains murmur and my zephyrs breathe;
> " Slow slides the painted snail—the gilded fly
> " Smooths his fine down to charm thy curious eye;
> " On twinkling fins my pearly nations play,
> " Or win with sinuous train their trackless way;
> " My plumy pairs in gay embroidery drest,
> " Form with ingenious bill the pensile nest,
> " To love's soft notes attune the listening dell,
> " And Echo sounds her soft symphonious shell."

And surely parents ought to coincide with their benign Creator, and permit them to enjoy for a few years the various delights he has prepared for them, and which appear almost necessary to their existence. The time will soon arrive when they must be confined to different studies and occupations, and then they will infalliby sicken and decay, unless the *mind* and *body* have both been duly invigorated, the one by early precept and admonition, the other by abundant exercise in sports and amusements such as all-wise Nature excites them to delight in.

The complexions of your daughters may be

as well guarded as you please from the rude effects of the elements: this done, let them run and enjoy themselves in full liberty, for a few hours every day, being properly attended by some faithful domestic, and they will inhale health and beauty from every breeze.

And as for your sons, let me entreat you to reflect upon what manner of men you will wish to see them in after life, and as you determine, so regulate your conduct now. Do you wish to see them effeminate and pusillanimous, then be it your care to guard their complexions, to instil into their tender minds the love of dress and show, to lead their attention to the best drest guest, and most splendid equipage—teach them to believe true excellence consists in sporting with superior grace the lily hand and diamond ring—

> " Betwixt the finger and the thumb to hold
> " The pouncet box"—

The poison will quickly pervade the whole soul of your children, and they will grow up the *things* you wish them. But if, on the other hand, you wish to rear the hero and the sage, teach them betimes to set no more than their just value on the trappings of fashion, the mere escutcheons to adorn, and set off to advantage the nobler part, altogether beneath the anxious notice of an immortal being, born to high honours, and capable of vast attainments. Teach them to exclaim with the gallant Hotspur—

> " By Heaven! methinks it were an easy leap
> " To pluck bright honour from the pale faced moon,
> " Or dive into the bottom of the deep,
> " Where fathom line could never touch the ground,
> " And pluck up drowned honour by the locks!
> " So he that doth redeem her thence, might wear
> " Without co-rival all her dignities."
>
> SHAKSPEARE.

At the same time that you insensibly instil into their youthful minds such just ideas of right and wrong, as shall " grow with their growth, and strengthen with their strength," enabling them through life to distinguish between that well earned *honour* which is at once the basis and reward of true courage and real merit, and that *air bubble* which owes its existence to the breath of the multitude, and which a rude puff may elevate on high or sink into insignificance, and from that barbarous, blood-thirsty sentiment, which aims the deadly weapon at the loved bosom of a darling, perhaps, an only friend.

But I am wandering beyond my bounds. Pardon, gentle reader, my zeal on this important subject, and impute it to the real and sole cause, a desire to promote the best interests of your lovely and beloved children.

I must now take my leave, with the sincere hope that this little volume may answer the end for which it is presented to the public, and assist the young and inexperienced mother in the discharge of duties, on the due fulfilment of which depend the future beauty, health, and happiness of the rising generation, and, eventually, the welfare of the community at large.

It will be observed, as respects the medical part of this work, I have confined myself chiefly to those disorders which few children escape, and every mother may be called upon o nurse and prescribe for; and, if I have in any material degree deviated from the most approved methods of treatment, I must beg the gentlemen of the faculty, if any such should honour my book with a perusal, to believe me open to conviction, and erring through ignorance or inexperience, not from vanity or empiricism.

NOTES.

NOTE (1), p. 170.

(Doses of Medicine adjusted to the Age.)

EVERY one knows that the doses of medicine should be adapted to different ages; but these are not in mere arithmetical or geometrical proportions, and their due relation is only to be ascertained by experience, and a reference to all the varieties of constitution and habits.

From the result of daily observation, one may say, for example, to a child of *seven years old, nearly half* the dose suitable for *adults;* to one of *three years,* the *fourth* part; of *one year,* the *sixth* part; and the *eighth* or *tenth* part to an infant in the *month*.

An adult person may take from fifteen to thirty grains of the testaceous powders, and double that quantity of magnesia, to be repeated two or three times a day; from fifteen to thirty grains of ipecacuanha, and from one to two of emetic tartar, as a vomit.

From one to two ounces of salts or of manna, and from ten to thirty grains of jalap, and from four to ten of calomel, as a purge. From ten to thirty drops of laudanum; the like number of grains of the extract of the white poppy, and from half an ounce to two ounces of its syrup as an anodyne: from this twofold direction, parents may perhaps attain to a more accurate estimation of the dose proper for their children, by the means of the experience they may have had of the particular quantity of any of the above medicines usually found sufficient for themselves whereinsoever that happens to vary from the dose here stated as proper for adults.

UNDERWOOD.

NOTE (2), p. 175.

Paregoric Elixir.

Take of acid, or flowers of benzoin, and saffron, of each	3 drachms.
Opium,	2 drachms.
Distilled Oil of Anise Seed,	½ a drachm.
Spirit of Ammonia, or Rectified Spirit,	2 pints.

Digest four days in a close vessel, then strain.

Edinburgh Dispensatory.

Elixir Proprietatis.

Take of Myrrh in Powder,	2 ounces.
Soccatrine Aloes,	1½ ounce.
Saffron,	1 ounce.
Rectified Spirit of Wine, Proof Spirit, of each	1 pound.

Digest the Myrrh with the Spirits four days, then add the aloes in powder, and the saffron; continue the digestion two days longer. Suffer the fæces to subside, and pour off the clear elixir.

Edinburgh Dispensatory.

This elixir I have found very efficacious for children afflicted with worms. Dose, ten or fifteen drops.

MEDICINES

RECOMMENDED IN THE DYSENTERY.

NOTE (3), p. 178.

Oil of Castor Emulsion.

Take Oil of Castor,	2 ounces.
Yolk of Egg, or Mucilage of Gum Arabic, sufficient to make it mix uniformly with Decoction of Barley,	10 ounces.
Syrup of Roses,	1 ounce.

Mix. Dose. Four table-spoonsful every second or third hour until the desired effect is obtained.

NOTE (4), p. 179.

Crystals of Tartar Whey.

Take Crystals of Tartar,	½ ounce.
Dissolve them in Milk,	½ a pint.
And add Manna,	2 ounces.

Infusion of Tamarinds.

Take Tamarinds,	1 ounce.
Boil them in Milk Whey,	8 ounces.
Then add Manna,	2 ounces.

Of each of these a tea-cupful or more may be taken occasionally.

Antiseptic Purging Apozem.

Take Tamarinds,	½ an ounce.
Boil them in water, from nine to seven ounces, then strain.	
Dissolve Manna,	2 ounces.
Tartarized Kali,	½ an ounce.
Mix.	

Antiseptic Aperient Draught.

Take Tartarized Kali,	40 grains.
Manna picked,	½ a drachm.
Lemon Juice,	2 drachms.
Distilled Water,	½ an ounce.

Mix. Any of these may be taken in proper doses, and repeated agreeably to the effect wanted to be produced.

WALLIS.

Sedative Fomentation.

Take the Heads of the White Poppy, bruised,	4 in number.
Let these be boiled in forty ounces of Water to twenty; then add,	
Vinegar	3 ounces.
Fixed Ammoniacal Salt,	5 drachms.
Mix.	

Nauseating Powder.

Take Ipecacuanha Powder,	1 grain.
Nitre, or Aromatic Powder,	10 grains.
To be taken every third hour.	

Decoction of Semirauba.

Take of Semirauba Bark,	2 drachms.
Distilled Water,	20 ounces, boiled to 16 ounces.

Dose. Four spoonsful.

MEDICINES

RECOMMENDED FOR THE MEASLES.

(See p. 199.)

Cooling Saline Purge.

Take Milk of Almonds, or Decoction of Barley,	10 ounces.
In which dissolve Vitriolated Natron,	1½ ounce.
Or Tartarized Natron,	1 ounce.
Or Vitriolated Kali,	½ an ounce.
Manna,	1 ounce.

Dose. Four table-spoonsful every third hour until the desired effect is produced.

Purging Draught.

Take infusion of Senna,	2 ounces.
Manna and Tincture of Senna, each,	½ an ounce.
Rhubarb in Powder,	8 or 10 grains.
Compound Spirit of Lavender,	2 drachms.

Mix.

OR,

Take Rhubarb, Jalap, in powder,	25 grains. 6 grains.
Cinnamon Water,	1 ounce.
Syrup of Orange Peel,	1 drachm.

Mix.

OR,

Take Rhubarb, in powder, 30 grains.

Mucilage of Gum Arabic, sufficient to form it into pills, or syrup may be added to make it into a bolus. Any of these forms may be taken in the morning early, and when they begin to operate, worked off with weak broth or thin gruel.

Oily Emulsion.

Take Oil of Sweet Almonds,	1 ounce.
Gum Arabic,	2 drachms.
Fine Sugar,	½ an ounce.
Mix these well together, then gradually add decoction of barley,	8 ounces.

Dose. Three or four spoonsful often in the day.

Oily Linctus.

Take Oil of Sweet Almonds,	1 ounce.
Gum Arabic,	3 drachms.
Syrup of Marshmallows,	1½ ounce.

Mix these well together. Dose. Two or three spoonsful often in the day; or it may be acidulated with a few drops of diluted vitriolic acid; or an ounce of syrup of lemon may be added.

MEDICINES

FOR THE HOOPING COUGH.

(See p. 213.)

Emetic Mixture.

Take Tartarized Antimony,	6 grains.
Distilled Water,	6 ounces.
Syrup of Saffron,	½ an ounce.

Mix. Dose. Two table-spoonsful repeated every half hour until the desired effect is produced.

Antimonial Mixture.

Take Tartarized Antimony,	3 grains.
Rose Water,	6 ounces.
Syrup of Sugar,	3 ounces.

Mix. Dose. One or two spoonsful every six or eight hours.

Saline Anodyne Draught.

Take Kali prepared,	10 grains.
Lemon Juice,	2 drachms.
Distilled Water,	1 ounce.
Tincture of Opium,	15 drops.
Syrup of White Poppy Heads,	2 drachms.

Mix. Dose as above.

The above medicines are all taken from Dr. Wallis's Treatise on the "Art of Preserving and Restoring Health," and are, therefore, presumed to be correct; but it must be remembered by my readers, that the doses are all calculated for adults, and must be proportioned according to the ages of the children to whom they are given. I shall now offer a recipe given me by a very skilful physician, who assured me of its efficacy, but as I have not tried it, having never seen a case of the hooping cough since it came into my possession, I cannot recommend it from experience; I have, however, great faith in the skill, and reliance upon the honour, of the gentleman who recommended the medicine, and, in the hope that it may prove beneficial, in some instances at least, I give it a place here.

CURE FOR THE HOOPING COUGH.

Dissolve a scruple of salt of tartar in a quarter of a pint of water, add to it ten grains of cochineal finely powdered, sweeten this with fine sugar, and give an infant a tea-spoonful four times a day. To a child of two or three years old two tea-spoonsful, from four years and upwards a table-spoonful or more may be taken. The relief is immediate, and the cure in general within five or six days.

FINIS.

Medicine & Society In America

An Arno Press/New York Times Collection

Alcott, William A. **The Physiology of Marriage.** 1866. New Introduction by Charles E. Rosenberg.

Beard, George M. **American Nervousness:** Its Causes and Consequences. 1881. New Introduction by Charles E. Rosenberg.

Beard, George M. **Sexual Neurasthenia.** 5th edition. 1898.

Beecher, Catharine E. **Letters to the People on Health and Happiness.** 1855.

Blackwell, Elizabeth. **Essays in Medical Sociology.** 1902. Two volumes in one.

Blanton, Wyndham B. **Medicine in Virginia in the Seventeenth Century.** 1930.

Bowditch, Henry I. **Public Hygiene in America.** 1877.

Bowditch, N[athaniel] I. **A History of the Massachusetts General Hospital:** To August 5, 1851. 2nd edition. 1872.

Brill, A. A. **Psychanalysis:** Its Theories and Practical Application. 1913.

Cabot, Richard C. **Social Work:** Essays on the Meeting-Ground of Doctor and Social Worker. 1919.

Cathell, D. W. **The Physician Himself and What He Should Add to His Scientific Acquirements.** 2nd edition. 1882. New Introduction by Charles E. Rosenberg.

The Cholera Bulletin. Conducted by an Association of Physicians. Vol. I: Nos. 1–24. 1832. All published. New Introduction by Charles E. Rosenberg.

Clarke, Edward H. **Sex in Education;** or, A Fair Chance for the Girls. 1873.

Committee on the Costs of Medical Care. **Medical Care for the American People:** The Final Report of The Committee on the Costs of Medical Care, No. 28. [1932].

Currie, William. **An Historical Account of the Climates and Diseases of the United States of America.** 1792.

Davenport, Charles Benedict. **Heredity in Relation to Eugenics.** 1911. New Introduction by Charles E. Rosenberg.

Davis, Michael M. **Paying Your Sickness Bills.** 1931.

Disease and Society in Provincial Massachusetts: Collected Accounts, 1736–1939. 1972.

Earle, Pliny. **The Curability of Insanity:** A Series of Studies. 1887.

Falk, I. S., C. Rufus Rorem, and Martha D. Ring. **The Costs of Medical Care:** A Summary of Investigations on The Economic Aspects of the Prevention and Care of Illness, No. 27. 1933.

Faust, Bernhard C. **Catechism of Health:** For the Use of Schools, and for Domestic Instruction. 1794.

Flexner, Abraham. **Medical Education in the United States and Canada:** A Report to The Carnegie Foundation for the Advancement of Teaching, Bulletin Number Four. 1910.

Gross, Samuel D. **Autobiography of Samuel D. Gross, M.D.,** with Sketches of His Contemporaries. Two volumes. 1887.

Hooker, Worthington. **Physician and Patient;** or, A Practical View of the Mutual Duties, Relations and Interests of the Medical Profession and the Community. 1849.

Howe, S. G. **On the Causes of Idiocy.** 1858.

Jackson, James. **A Memoir of James Jackson, Jr., M.D.** 1835.

Jennings, Samuel K. **The Married Lady's Companion, or Poor Man's Friend.** 2nd edition. 1808.

The Maternal Physician; a Treatise on the Nurture and Management of Infants, from the Birth until Two Years Old. 2nd edition. 1818. New Introduction by Charles E. Rosenberg.

Mathews, Joseph McDowell. **How to Succeed in the Practice of Medicine.** 1905.

McCready, Benjamin W. **On the Influences of Trades, Professions, and Occupations in the United States, in the Production of Disease.** 1943.

Mitchell, S. Weir. **Doctor and Patient.** 1888.

Nichols, T[homas] L. **Esoteric Anthropology:** The Mysteries of Man. [1853].

Origins of Public Health in America: Selected Essays, 1820–1855. 1972.

Osler, Sir William. **The Evolution of Modern Medicine.** 1922.

The Physician and Child-Rearing: Two Guides, 1809–1894. 1972.

Rosen, George. **The Specialization of Medicine:** with Particular Reference to Ophthalmology. 1944.

Royce, Samuel. **Deterioration and Race Education.** 1878.

Rush, Benjamin. **Medical Inquiries and Observations.** Four volumes in two. 4th edition. 1815.

Shattuck, Lemuel, Nathaniel P. Banks, Jr., and Jehiel Abbott. **Report of a General Plan for the Promotion of Public and Personal Health.** Massachusetts Sanitary Commission. 1850.

Smith, Stephen. **Doctor in Medicine** and Other Papers on Professional Subjects. 1872.

Still, Andrew T. **Autobiography of Andrew T. Still,** with a History of the Discovery and Development of the Science of Osteopathy. 1897.

Storer, Horatio Robinson. **The Causation, Course, and Treatment of Reflex Insanity in Women.** 1871.

Sydenstricker, Edgar. **Health and Environment.** 1933.

Thomson, Samuel. **A Narrative, of the Life and Medical Discoveries of Samuel Thomson.** 1822.

Ticknor, Caleb. **The Philosophy of Living;** or, The Way to Enjoy Life and Its Comforts. 1836.

U.S. Sanitary Commission. **The Sanitary Commission of the United States Army:** A Succinct Narrative of Its Works and Purposes. 1864.

White, William A. **The Principles of Mental Hygiene.** 1917.